FITTER AFTER 50

Forever Changing Our Beliefs About Aging

By

Ed Mayhew with Mary Mayhew

ISBN: 1-4033-0256-1 (e-book)
ISBN: 1-4033-0257-X (Paperback)
ISBN: 1-4033-0258-8 (Dustjacket)

This book is printed on acid free paper.

1st Books - rev. 06/20/02

Dedication

Dedicated to
All the Masters of Fitness who are showing us that we can
indeed be Fitter After 50

TABLE OF CONTENTS

Acknowledgements

First, I thank our Masters of Fitness, who in choosing to be fitter after 50 have shown us that we can, too. They generously gave of their time to answer my questions and share their secrets. My sincere appreciation, friendship, and feelings of awe go out to:

Payton Jordan, Ruth Anderson (and Dick Collins), Norm Green, Jean Sterling, Warren Utes, June Tatro, Helen Klein, Carl Kristenson, Ken Morrison, Denver and Nora Fox, James Hill, Jerry Dunn, Pat Rice, and Janet Baker-Murray. These are champions all — most of all, Champions of Life.

Another group that has helped me and will help you are the pioneers of fitness. These individuals have done the research and designed the programs that work. Their expertise, which they so generously share, is a blessing to us all:

Dr. Philip Maffetone, Bill Phillips, Kenneth E. Cooper, M.D., Glenn A. Gaessar, Ph.D., Doc Lew Childre, Miriam E. Nelson, Ph.D., and John A. McDougall, M.D.

Some local heroes of fitness represent the tens of thousands across the country and the world who are examples of what is possible post 50:

Burr Grim, Randy Wingfield, Sandy Adams, Chuck Raper, Ray Kitchen, Ray Gordon, Kathy Smart, and Jason Page.

More thanks go to:

Garth Battista of Breakaway Books (BreakAwayBooks.com); Jan Seeley of *Marathon and Beyond* magazine (MarathonAndBeyond.com); and Columnist Bard Lindeman, *The Bard of Aging* (BeOutrageous.com) for giving me permission to use quotes from their publications.

Charles Henderson, Christian Kelly, and the folks at First Books Library for publishing *FA50*.

Richard Kerby and Karston Brown, Shenandoah Valley Runners (SVRunners.org) for allowing me to quote him (Rick) and giving me contact with the local fitness heroes.

Jerry and Esther Hicks whose work illumines these writings and ties it all together. For more information about the art of allowing fitness and all manner of well-being into your life go to Abraham-Hicks.com.

All of you I inadvertently forgot to name — Thank You!

My daughter, Joanna, for helping with the manuscript and some computer glitches.

Keith Boyd for his computer expertise and willingness to help.

My wife, Mary, who rightfully accuses me of gleefully sprinkling a salt shakerful of commas willy-nilly over every page of my work. Thanks to her editing, you will be spared my mangled modifiers, calamitous clauses, and the dangling of my participles.

Finally, my heartfelt appreciation to you for purchasing/reading *FA50*. May your beliefs about aging be forever changed and may you be fitter after 50.

INTRODUCTION

You may have some questions:

- Can we *really* be fitter after 50?
- Fitter than what?
- What is your definition of fitter?
- Do I truly need or want to be more fit?
- Isn't aging natural and inevitable?
- How is *Fitter After 50* different from the myriad diet, exercise, and other self-improvement books already glutting the market?
- Who is Ed Mayhew?
- Isn't getting fitter after 50 going to be awfully hard to do?
- How much is it going to cost?
- Will this be time consuming?
- Aren't there ...

J.Q.: Can we *really* be fitter after 50?

Mayhew: In my research and interviews I found countless individuals, male and female, who are definitely fitter after 50. Their stories are fascinating, inspiring, and the centerpiece of *FA50*. Some were veritable couch potatoes before their metamorphosis; some had disease conditions to overcome; others were already fit to begin with; but all of them are certifiably fitter after 50. For example, Gerry Davidson has just set a world record for 80-year-old women with a 9-minute-flat mile run. It's safe to say that 95 percent or more of our 20-year-olds cannot run a mile that fast; many of them can't run a mile, period! Septuagenarian Ed Whitlock just missed breaking the 3-hour barrier for a marathon by 25 seconds. That's a seventy-year-old averaging under 7 minutes per mile for 26 miles. It is a rare 20 or 30-year-old who can run a *single* 6-plus-minute mile. Want more proof? When Anson "Clappy" Clapcott took up running in 1990 he finished dead last in a 5 miler. A year later, in his second race, he finished last again. In 2001, Anson at age 56 WON the Tybee (Ga.) Marathon with a time of 2:47:25.

J.Q.: Fitter than what?

Mayhew: The 50 to 90-plus-year-olds you'll meet in this book are fitter than the average 40-year-old; most are fitter than the majority of those in their thirties; and many are more fit than even the typical 20-something. The vast majority are fitter than they themselves were before crossing the half-century mark. In a way, they have actually turned back the biological hands of time.

J.Q.: That's nice, but just what is your definition of fitter?

Mayhew: For this book's discussion, fitter means stronger, leaner, and healthier with more endurance, flexibility, agility, vibrancy and energy. As you meet these extraordinary people of *FA50*, you will come to realize that they are all these qualities and more. Their accomplishments will blow you away and let you know just how much more the human mind/body is capable of accomplishing than we realize. We assume that our bodies get frail with age, but we will see that this just doesn't *need* to be so. Not at all!

J.Q.: Do I truly need or want to be more fit?

Mayhew: Well, most people after age 25 (those who don't take steps to get or stay fit) lose 5 pounds of muscle each decade and usually replace them with fat. Researcher/author, Miriam E. Nelson, Ph.D., says that women typically lose about 2 percent of their *muscle* strength each year. Other research shows that we lose about 30 percent of our muscle mass between young adulthood and old age. Let's say we are a typical, slender 20-year-old male weighing 150 pounds with a mere 10 percent bodyfat. That means that as a young adult we would have only 15 pounds of bodyfat. That's good! Now let's say we arrive at age 55 (after 35 years of an ever increasing sedentary lifestyle) still weighing just 150 pounds. You would probably say that's good — maintaining the same weight over the years. But alas, now you are 33% fat, or to put it another way — 50 pounds of unadulterated lard. You now have 35 more pounds of fat (50 take away 15) to be lugged around by 35 fewer pounds of muscle. No wonder we don't have the pep and energy of youth. But wait; it gets worse. If you *gained* any weight over the years it would not be muscle (unless you've done something to build muscle, which in our typical scenario you haven't). Therefore, if your weight has increased a measly 10 pounds to 160, that's an additional 10 pounds of fat or a total of 60 pounds of adipose tissue to cart around all day. But what if you had ballooned to a nice even 200 pounds? In this case, you are now one-half fat; 100 pounds of you is lean, fat-burning tissue and the other 100 pounds is just stored fat which is putting added stress on your arthritic joints, your heart and blood vessels, and your initiative to get up, get going, and enjoy life to the fullest.

Why be fitter after 50? If you don't, sooner or later you'll have to give up some of the things you love. Things like picking up your grandchildren, giving them piggyback rides up to bed, playing tag or ball, ... Eventually you will have to give up some of your other loves, such as golfing, hunting, shopping, traveling, driving, getting out of your chair, getting off the toilet without help, etc. But by being fitter, we can delay or prevent this unwelcome day's arrival. Put another way, while some 75-year-olds are traveling across the country and the world, visiting with friends and family and even skiing or scuba diving, others 75 and younger are in nursing homes needing help to dress, feed themselves, and tend to their most basic bodily functions. There are simple, easy steps we can take to see that we greatly increase the odds that we will be enjoying life right up to the end.

There is also the issue of not being a burden on our children — financially, physically or emotionally. Financially speaking, the cost of not taking care of ourselves is staggering. Healthcare in the U.S. is at about 15% of gross national product. That's more than any other industrialized country. Those over 65 pay an average of $12,000 per year for healthcare; for those over 85 it is an astronomical $20,000. This can easily wipe out a retirement nest egg and leave our children and grandchildren holding the bag, directly or indirectly (through stifling increases in taxes to pay for the healthcare needs of the elderly).

J.Q.: Isn't aging natural and inevitable?

Mayhew: Yes, aging is natural and unpreventable if your definition of aging is getting older chronologically, but the number of years one has been on the planet Earth is just a number that has been assigned to determine passage of time.

Biological aging is another thing altogether and although it sometimes entails getting diseased, feeble, and falling down a lot, those maladies are not part and parcel of biological aging. BA deals with biological signs or markers in the body, such as loss of muscle, a slowing metabolism, and rising blood pressure. However, a slowing metabolism and the resulting middle-age spread are not genetically preordained; neither are high-blood pressure, sky-rocketing cholesterol, arthritic joints, adult-onset diabetes, osteoporosis, heart disease and strokes. These are all the result of, or exacerbated by, poor lifestyle choices and will be addressed in a later chapter.

Some boomers are actually becoming biologically younger. Their markers for aging are reverting to more youthful levels. For instance, their muscle mass, which typically shrinks with age, is increasing; their metabolism is speeding up to youthful levels; and their bone density is on the rebound. Miriam Nelson, Ph.D., reports in her landmark Tufts University strength training study, published in the Journal of the American Medical Association, that "We found *that* after a year of strength training twice a week, older women's bodies were 15 to 20 years younger."

Likewise, Dean Ornish, M.D., has shown that heart disease can actually be reversed using natural means. Numerous other individuals have successfully eliminated, or greatly reduced their need for, high blood pressure, cholesterol, and other medications with the help of John McDougall, M.D. and his program. Deepak Chopra, M.D., renowned author and lecturer, on his web site says it well, "Modern science has shown that many of the most important biological markers of aging can be reversed through your interpretation and lifestyle changes."

Again, you will be meeting, in *FA50,* ordinary folks like yourself who have, to one degree or another, reversed the aging process. I will also be sharing some fitness programs that have been successful in slowing, halting, or even reversing the aging process.

J.Q.: How is *Fitter After 50* different from the unending parade of diet, exercise, and other self-improvement books in the marketplace?

Mayhew: Most of the other books are How-To Books, whereas *FA50* is more of a Why-To Book, an If-They-Can-Do-It-

I-Can-Do-It Book, and a This-Is-Where-You-Can-Find-It Book. The "If-They-Can-Do-It-I-Can-Do-It" stories of Master fitness champs/Senior athletes of all ages, backgrounds, and beginning places will develop a rock-solid belief that you really can be fitter after 50. The "whys" will strengthen your desire and resolve. The "where-tos" will take you to proven, effective, easy-to-follow fitness programs. This is not just another How-To-Book; it's a paper-and-ink personal trainer that will get you started and keep you going on the path to a fitter, happier you.

We know we should eat better and get more exercise, ..., but life keeps getting in the way of our noble intentions. We either procrastinate and never get started or we run out of gas after a few days or weeks of being "good." The name of the game is consistency and *FA50* gives you everything you need to get started and stick with it for the long haul. You can, and I'll show you *how*. (whoops!)

J.Q.: Who is this Ed Mayhew guy?

Mayhew: A lifetime of study, research (including dozens of interviews with the Masters of Fitness for *FA50*), and life experience in the fitness arena makes me uniquely qualified to share this message of hope. In addition I have a B.A. degree in health and fitness and 35 years of teaching experience in this arena (and I have a couple of books on this subject to my credit). I don't come to you with piles of degrees and pedigrees to hide behind or use as a pedestal to prop myself up. I'm content to be judged on my words, message, and deeds. You won't be disappointed.

J.Q.: Isn't getting fitter after 50 going to be hard?

Mayhew: The good news is that the more sedentary and less fit you are the easier it is to see and experience dramatic results in a relatively short time (days or weeks) with minimal effort. The better the shape you are in, the harder it is to improve, but in that case you already are fitter than most. Just a few pounds dropped, as an example, can improve your blood pressure, blood sugar and cholesterol numbers.

J.Q.: How much is it going to cost?

Mayhew: The real question is: what is it going to cost if you don't? Your independence? Your health? Your enjoyment of life? It is not unusual for Seniors to drop one or two thousand dollars each year on prescription drugs. On the other hand, one can drastically improve his life through simple lifestyle changes without spending much at all.

J.Q.: Won't this be too time consuming?

Mayhew: Actually, you'll create more time to do the things you like and need to do because you'll have more energy to get your tasks and work done quicker. This will give you more time, not less, for family, friends, and leisure pursuits.

J.Q.: My Aunt Erma is 97 and never exercised a day in her life and she has a rotten diet and a worse attitude!

Mayhew: We're looking at improving the quality of our life, not just the length. Spending the last 10 years of one's life in a nursing home vegetating like some potted plant is not exactly what we want. There are so many variables that affect one's health that we can't say exactly why one person lives to a ripe, old 107, while another leaves us at 74. We are playing with odds here. We want to stack the deck in our favor for a fun, enjoyable life, for however long we live.

Fitter after 50 is intended for healthy adults. This book is solely for informational and educational purposes and is not medical advice. Please consult a medical or health professional before you begin any new exercise, nutrition, supplementation, or lifestyle-change program or if you have questions about your health. The individuals featured in this book have achieved extraordinary results; there are no "typical" results. Their success stories represent extraordinary examples of what can be accomplished through an integrated system of exercise, nutrition, and belief. As individuals differ, their results will differ, even when using the same or similar programs.

CHAPTER 1 FITTER AFTER 50 WHYS

Most of us know that we *should* be exercising on a regular basis, eating well and otherwise taking care of ourselves. So why do so few do it? Why are 50 or 60 percent (depending on which study is cited) of us overweight? Why are high blood pressure, diabetes, arthritis, heart disease, cancers and other degenerative diseases rampant? More important, why do some stick with their workouts and healthful diets while most fall back into their unhealthy ways or never seem to get started in the first place?

The answer is quite simple. We have to really believe that all that sweat and fuss is going to make a measurable difference in the way we feel, look, and function. Secondly, we have to have a strong desire to change. We are very comfortable in the status quo, thank you very much, despite the daily misery it brings us. We must build the desire to get out of our chair, off the couch, out from in front of the computer/TV screen — out of these comfort zones. We really are comfortable where we are; *even* if it includes a certain amount of boredom, discomfort and YES, even pain. That is why, despite the lack of energy, rolls of fat, the threatening cholesterol levels, the impending chronic diseases (present or future), the poor self-image, the nagging thoughts that we should get back in shape, and the general malaise, we fail to take action to improve our lot. Lastly, we need a plan — a program that we can follow that we believe, or better yet, know will work for us.

This chapter deals with the desire issue. We have to have a good reason to get up off of our fatty acids and start sweating like a pig; not to mention trading in some of our comforting food friends for a healthier fare. Well, deprivation and Spartan-like exercise routines seldom work for long. We don't recommend either one of them, but we are getting ahead of ourselves. Right now, we will deal just with building our desire; for when desire is strong enough (and belief is rock solid), we take action and the progress is lasting and the results are breathtaking. Also, when there is a burning desire, the "how" will take care of itself (again, another chapter).

1

If we are to make lasting changes that will result in our looking our best, feeling terrific, and performing optimally both physically as well as mentally, then we must stoke the fire of desire. With that in mind, here are fifty reasons to revamp our lifestyle so that we really can be fitter after 50.

Some of these "whys" are serious, others silly and just plain off the wall. Read them as if you wrote them yourself. In other words, when "I" is used, it refers to you. They are meant to stimulate thought and fire up your desire to be fitter after 50. If they provoke other divergent ideas, you might want to jot them down for later rumination. If one hits home, makes you cringe, laugh, or say, "Yes!", then you may want to mark it for later review. In chapter 4 we will look at some mental exercises where you can use these "whys" for inspiration. Without further ado, here they are in no particular order. Enjoy!

I Want To Be Fitter After 50 Because ...
1. Fitter after 50 beats fatter after 50 hands down.
2. Life is better when we have the energy to enjoy our evenings with our family and friends instead of just crashing on the couch.
3. Sometimes in an emergency, we have to be able to move fast (or lift and carry) in order to save ourselves, a loved one, or a coworker.
4. For some Seniors the simple act of sitting down on the toilet and then getting back up again can be a real challenge. Having to call 911 on our cell phone and then having the local rescue squad break down the bathroom door to find us on the pot is a harrowing thought for some of us. Don't let this happen to you!
5. Long-term healthcare is expensive, can drag on for twelve years and more, and has been known to wipe out life savings. By staying in top shape, we can avoid, delay, or lessen this emotionally and financially draining situation.
6. I hear that life is better (and healthier, too) when our chest is bigger than our belly.
7. I don't want some doctor to tell me that I *have* to give up the foods that I love.

8. The alternative, sooner or later, is likely to involve taking prescription medicines for the rest of my life (for a chronic heart condition or ...) — with their expense and unpleasant side effects.

9. Hearing your doctor say, at the end of a complete physical, that you have the body of someone 20 years younger — and you are going to have to give it back.

It Is My Intention To Be Fitter After 50 Because ...

10. I don't want to *ever* have to give up my favorite hobbies and activities — such as, golfing, gardening, and skiing.

11. It is better to pick wildflowers with a loved one than to push them up by yourself.

12. I don't know about you, but the idea of a surgeon needing to pry open my chest to perform open heart surgery is not a pleasant thought.

13. Looking 80 when you are 60 is not quite as much fun as looking 40 when you are really 60.

14. The pimply stockboy at the supermarket has just proudly placed the last can on the 6-foot pyramid of peas. As he wipes his brow and takes a moment to admire the fruits of his hour of toil, you reach for some canned goods on a nearby shelf. Suddenly, due to a lack of strength in your aged legs, you lose your balance and — you guessed it — end up sitting in a sea of dented cans of peas.

15. Having to give up traveling to fun and interesting places would be a real shame.

16. I want to be able to enjoy playing ball with my grandchildren and great-grandchildren.

17. When that "punk" teen calls me "pops" I can challenge him to a game of hoops and "whoop his butt" (his terminology, of course).

18. When traveling across the country with my children and their families and we stop at a scenic overlook, I don't want to have to stay with the vehicle and miss all the fun because I can't walk the 500 feet uphill to the overlook or

3

negotiate the rugged-mile trail to a spectacular waterfall.

19. One day you wake up and realize that if it weren't for an ocassional bowel movement, you wouldn't be getting any exercise at all.

I Am Making The Decision To Be Fitter After 50 Because ...

20. I want to enjoy the accolades one gets when completing a marathon for the first time! I will revel in doing that which my friends and family think I am too old to do.

21. It will be fun to meet people I know at the beach or pool, while partaking of the water activities, and have them comment on how great I look (in jaw-dropping fashion).

22. I would love to hear my healthcare professional say, "In all my 30 years of practicing medicine I've never seen anyone your age with such good _____."

23. Your grandchild has wandered into the street and a big truck is coming. You realize that if you could only run, just a little, you could save him.

24. I don't want to have to explain to my grandson why Santa Claus was too weak, tired, or drunk on eggnog from around the world to hang up his stocking when he finds it (with its 25-pound payload) lying on the floor at the foot of the fireplace mantle with telltale "drag marks" the length of the livingroom rug.

25. The sheer joy of having family and friends cheering for me at the finish line and along the course of a long-distance biking, running or swimming race would be a hoot.

26. A friend or family member desperately needs my support, presence, or help and I am physically able to drive the 500 miles/10 hours to be there for him in his hour of need.

27. It is never too late to get in shape! And, the worse shape one is in the less effort it takes to make dramatic gains.

28. Otherwise, because of my lack of fitness and/or poor health, I could have to pay ten thousand dollars to have someone else build a porch that I could have built myself (AND built better) if I had only stayed in better shape.

29. I could recreate some of the youthful gyrations in the backseat of a Chevy, Ford, or Lamborginni, ... AND not get excruciating cramps in my back, legs, neck, etc.

I Am Committing To Being Fitter After 50 Because ...

30. I can imagine how much fun it would be to enter a 10k (6.2 miles) foot race and finish in the front of the pack (the first third) and see teenagers, 20-year-olds, and 30-somethings finishing after me.

31. When you've taken a second mortgage on the house to take your grandchild to *the* theme park of all theme parks and he's moaning, whining and miserable from walking too much, you can easily hoist him up onto your back for a fun piggyback ride without *your* silently moaning, whining, and being miserable.

32. When I Know that I have been eating and exercising well (I've been "good"), I can afford to *sin* a little and treat myself to that rich, decadent dessert that I love — without feeling any guilt or doing any "damage."

33. By strengthening my muscles and improving my circulation I can better protect my hip and knee joints so that a hip or knee replacement is not a part of my future.

34. Putting together my eager kindergarten-age grandchild's indoor fort (all 1,043 pieces with directions by an illiterate Taiwanese with an attitude) *without* turning red, perspiring heavily and then inconveniently croaking right in front of little Johnnie (thus ruining, by neuro-association, all his birthdays for the rest of his miserable, guilt-filled life) would be good.

35. I would love to have the fitness level needed to finally do that skydiving, scuba diving, or race-car driving that I have always wanted to do.
36. The prospect of saving my cash-strapped son tons of money by helping shingle his leaks-like-a-sieve roof — a rigorous, 2 day/all day job excites me.
37. Being able to get down on the floor to play with my grandchildren *and* to be able to get back up again the same day would be nifty.
38. It would feel good to have the superior fitness and abundance of time (due to being retired) to be able help search on foot, in rugged territory, for that lost toddler (who's the same age as my only grandchild) whose plight was broadcast on the local news. I can imagine the thrill of being part of a successful rescue effort, like this, that returns the youngster to his family unharmed.
39. Row 5 at a Wayne Newton concert is better than a front row seat at the Shady Pines for the singing of "I Gotta Be Me" by a guy named LeRoy who's only claim to fame is a second place finish at the regional Kariyoke Singalong in 1987.

I Choose To Be Fitter After 50 Because ...
40. It is easier and less expensive to get new parts for my car than it is to get them for my body.
41. I can imagine the feeling when, for the first time in twenty-some years, I am able to slip into a size ____ dress.
42. I would like to dance the night away like I did in the old days, without needing the medics to later come and cart me away.
43. Cancelling travel plans to visit friends or family because the cost of medicines/prescriptions/surgeries (even with insurance and/or medicare) has wiped out the travel funds, would be depressing.
44. Two times a night ain't so bad when it changes from referring to how many times you get up in

the night to go to the bathroom to how many amorous encounters you have.

45. You know you are old when putting on your clothes becomes the major part of your morning, as well as the highlight.

46. I don't want to wake up some time in the future to find that the best part of my days on the raisin ranch is waiting to be changed twice a day and having my bottom powdered.

47. One day, I want to be able to ask my husband if these Jeans "make my butt look too big," knowing that he no longer has to lie to keep the peace and fully appreciating the sincerity of his compliment.

48. I want to be fitter after 50 because it is plain FUN!

49. During a night of particularly amorous sheet rustling, you get stuck in the "docking position." Due to a combination of arthritis, leg cramps, and just plain stiff joints, you are unable to extricate yourselves and the National Guard has to be called out to pry you apart with the jaws of life. Don't laugh, it could happen to you!

50. I choose to be fitter after 50 because **I CAN!**

50.5 Being fitter after 50 means I can _____
_____

Using these fifty "whys" to stimulate and expand your thinking, make a list of *your* most compelling reasons. You can create as many reasons to be fitter after 50 as you would like, but then select the five most pertinent to you — the ones that are most likely to drive you to take consistent, daily and weekly, action. Write these down below and use them with some of the empowering techniques in chapter 4 that will lock in lifelong attitudes and behaviors for a fitter you after 50!

  1. _____
  2. _____
  3. _____
  4. _____
  5. _____

In the next two chapters we are going to meet some ordinary folks, just like you and me, whose fitness feats are of legendary proportions and who have blazed the trail to a fitter-after-50 tomorrow for all of us.

CHAPTER 2 IF THEY CAN DO IT ...
THE YOUNGSTERS — 50s & 60s

We want to look good, feel great, and function well. We desire robust health, bounding energy, and a strong, graceful body right into old age. So why don't we do something to make these desires a reality? The truth is, we don't believe we can have the boundless energy of youth, the streamlined body, the vitality or we believe the price would be too great.

As long as we feel that nothing we do would make a significant-enough difference or we see the cost in time and effort as exorbitant or futile, we'll do nothing, or just give a half-hearted effort.

But what if you *knew* that vibrant well-being could be yours again with minimal exertion on your part. The stronger your belief that this is true, that you can make dramatic changes in self for the better, the easier it is to take action — significant action that will actually transform your life.

The individuals you are about to meet in this chapter and chapter 3 will make you say to yourself, "If they can do it, then I can too! If 75-year-old great-grandmother, Helen Klein, can run a 100-mile race, then surely I can start a regular 30-minute walking or running program. If Peter Jurczyk, at 91, can swim a mile at a time during his training sessions, then I can get the exercise I need. If Carl Kristenson can enter his first body-building competition at age 55, then maybe I can get in decent enough shape so that I don't embarrass myself when I walk on the beach or frighten myself when I get out of the tub and see my reflection in the full-length mirror."

The object here is not to get you to run 100 miles, swim competitively, or enter body-building contests. I can hear you now, "That'll be the day!!" It is just to show you what is possible; and just how remarkably fit 50- and-60-year-old-and-older bodies/individuals can become. Bent over, slow moving, stiff, using a walker, and becoming ever more frail are not the result of aging; they **are the result of poor lifestyle choices** in many if not most cases.

You will find mostly runners in this chapter and book because just about anyone can identify with someone running differing numbers of miles. You have some experience with running different distances during your youth or as an adult chasing a bus, for example; and you are familiar with distances, such as 1 or 10 miles. So when we say someone has run 5 miles or 50 miles, you can relate it to your own experiences and think, "How in the world can anyone ....." On the other hand, it is not quite so clear how much effort a 90-year-old tennis player is exerting. Also, due to the simplicity of running (one foot in front of the other over and over again), and the low costs involved (all one really needs is a good pair of running shoes), etc., there are more senior runners to study than senior football players or senior hang-glider enthusiasts. We are not necessarily promoting long-distance running over any other aerobic activity, but rather giving you something to which you can relate.

When you finish this chapter, you will know in your heart that you can greatly improve your lot in life. You will no longer buy into the idea that aging means an inevitable and steady physical and mental decline. You will believe, again, that you truly are in control of your own destiny.

Here are some terms, as they are applied in *FA50*, to help you:

• The 5K is a 5 kilometer (3.1 Miles) footrace, bike race, etc.

• The 10K is a 10 kilometer (6.2 miles) race.

• A marathon is a race just over 26 miles in length.

• An ultra-marathon (also called an ultra) is any race longer than a marathon (e.g., 50K or 31 miles; 100K or 62 miles; 100 miles; 24-hour race or how far can travel in 24 hours; and a 6-day race or how far can travel in, you got it, 6 days).

• WAVA — World Association of Veteran Athletes (in 2001 changed name to World Masters Athletics — WMA)

• Masters are athletes 40 or older. In races individuals can win or place in the masters division i.e., competing against others of a similar age; Senior masters are age 50 and older.

Chubby To Muscular In Just 45 Years

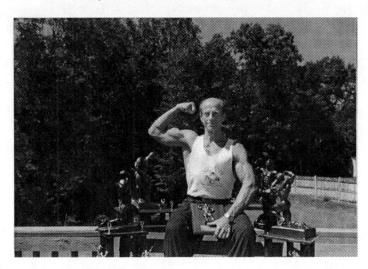

In 1994, at age 55, when too many of us are starting to wind down, **Carl Kristenson** decided to enter his first bodybuilding contest. Just imagine yourself standing on stage in just a skimpy bathing suit with strangers and friends alike ogling and analyzing your every physical attribute. For most of us, in our 50s or thereabouts, it would not be a pretty picture or a confidence-enhancing experience. However, for Carl, now 61, we can see by his body-building titles, finishes, and more, that this was a good move: Overall Champion in the Massachusetts Natural (no steroids or other artificial ingredients) Championships (GrandMasters — over 45-years-old); Overall Champion in the Maine Natural Championships (GrandMasters); Fifth in the United States Championships Over Age 50; and Fifth in the Over 60 Mr. America — to name a few.

Not bad for a "chubby kid" who grew up to struggle with his weight most of his adult life. Carl actually topped out at 212 pounds on a 5 foot 7 inch frame, and it wasn't all muscle.

When Carl set out to build his body he was in "fair shape" and weighed in at 174 pounds. With the help of a personal trainer, and a combination of weight training, cardiovascular work (fast walking), and diet he surprised himself by consistently dropping 2 pounds per week for 12 weeks. This put him at a muscular 150 pounds for his first competition — a third place in the Cape Cod Natural-GrandMasters.

What drove Carl when training became difficult, as it invariably does when one is competing with others at an elite level for a single prize? Carl says, "My motivation came from many areas: supreme effort and self-denial came from upcoming bodybuilding shows, but at age 55, health and physical appearance became very important." He goes on to say that, "over the counter supplements played a small part in my quest for physical excellence, so I suppose my approach was eclectic — a combination of any and all pertinent things that could help — except steroids or any other illegal aid. I am lifetime drug-free, a position reinforced by a strong Christian commitment."

Again, for Carl, motivation was the key. Knowledge of diet and exercise protocol supplied by experts and his personal trainer were critical, "but focus or mindset provided the consistency necessary to continue through the down times."

What, if anything, did Carl get from this laserbeam-like focus and intent, other than the trophies and titles? He received respect from peers, as well as younger folks, as they stood in awe of his accomplishments and obvious superior muscularity. It led to the fulfillment of a desire he had had to become an American Council on Exercise (ACE) certified personal trainer. He was given a platform from which to share his faith with young bodybuilders. Carl also gained a closer connection with his grandson — the Massachusetts State Champion in the javelin — and made many new friends while traveling throughout the Eastern United States.

What is Carl's advice for us? As seniors we should obviously get our doctor's approval before starting an exercise program or making major lifestyle changes, but even then we should proceed cautiously, "listening" to our bodies. If we can afford a personal trainer, we should get one. If not, read *sensible* materials about exercise and diet and stay away from those gimmicks seen on endless TV infomercials. No matter what fitness equipment you do or don't have, optimum results don't come from 5-minutes-a-day on this contraption or that state-of-the-art gizmo, but rather from consistency, dedication, hard work, and discipline. In conclusion he says, "There is no easy (lazy) way to optimum results. Motivation is a key ..."

Finally, I asked Carl if someone 50 or older can get or be in better shape than the *average* 20-to-30-year-old. Carl's response, "Absolutely! With hard work and dedication the average 50-year-old can get in *much* better shape than the *average* 20-to-30-year-old who isn't commited to health and fitness; and a 50-year-old who isn't 'in shape' can get in excellent condition with the proper program and motivation!"

If Carl can change from chubby to muscular to the point that at 55 and 60 he can outperform 45-and-50-year-old bodybuillders (as well as most young people), then "I" can transform my carcass, such as it is, into a work of art (and we don't mean a Picasso). We now know that if we expend some focused effort, we can once again walk down the beach and turn some heads AND for the right reasons!

7 Continents In 267 Days

If you met 50-year-old junior high school social studies teacher, **Brent Weigner**, on the street, the words "World Champion" would not come to mind. Yet, this unassuming, 3-time cancer survivor holds the world record for running an ultra-marathon on every continent (that's 7 for those of you who dozed off during social studies class) over a span of 267 days. Brent is a world-class athlete, often finishing his ultras among the top half dozen finishers overall and as the first-place American. He has also completed over 100 marathons.

What is Brent's motivation? He thrives on looking for new, unthought-of challenges; loves to travel; and enjoys the challenge, as well as, the act of running itself. His running "hobby" has given him an excuse to travel to 80 countries and most of the US states. In one race, the Inca Trail Ultra (more like an adventure run) where runners climb from 6,000 to 12,000 feet in the mountains of Peru, Brent came in third even though he ran an extra mile or two when he got lost.

As I see it, the keys to his success are:
1. Although he's gotten good results on only 3 or 4 hours of sleep the night prior to a big event, he's found that getting sufficient sleep the week before a race is crucial.
2. The high-altitude training in his hometown of Cheyenne, Wyoming gives him an advantage.
3. Including one long run every 10 to 14 days during training is critical, as is tapering down the amount of running in the days before a race.

13

4. During ultras he has found that consuming 100 to 200 calories per hour (mostly carbohydrates) and drinking 16 to 32 ounces of liquids during that same time period is imperative to replenish his glycogen stores (energy source stored in the muscles and liver) and stay hydrated. He thinks in terms of recovery *during* the race by drinking and eating even when not thirsty or hungry.

5. At the end of a day's run protein becomes essential so that muscle doesn't get metabolized (used as an energy source); during the event protein intake is not that important.

6. Brent doesn't want to think of running as a second job or to do it for the prize money; his inspiration comes from the challenge and the intrinsic joy-of-running itself.

7. He listens to his body, and depending on how his training is going and his emotional attachment to the race, decides whether to run as a competitor or just to finish the race. Brent has found that when he races hard, "the chances of seriously breaking down are enormously magnified."

If Brent, a 50-year-old teacher, can travel to the four corners of the world running ultra-marathons, then maybe we can hike the state and federal parks in our area of the country or we can ...

Turning Disaster Into Triumph

What would you do if your wife died leaving you with 3 young children to raise; and then you lost your job a few days later? If your name is **Terry Hitchcock**, you carry on as best you can raising your children; and then when the kids are older (10 years later) you create the Save The Children Foundation and plan a 2,000-mile run to raise funds and awareness to get the Foundation (for children who have lost their mothers) off the ground. So Terry set out to run the equivalent of 75 marathons in 75 days to promote his cause. The only trouble was he was in his fifties; had only run two 10K races, in both of which he had finished dead last; and he had a sore right achilles tendon that didn't allow him to take more than 5 or 6 mile training runs at a time. Then, six months into his 4 to 8 hours-per-day training (weights, flexibility exercises, and running), he had a heart attack. Despite the trials, tribulations and setbacks, with his doctor's blessing and his resolve strenghtened by the adversity, on May 2, 1996 Terry set out to run from Minneapolis-St. Paul to Atlanta, Georgia to raise funds and cognizance for his fledgling foundation.

The 56-year-old found the road to Atlanta paved with one hardship after another, from a first month filled with rain and abnormally cold weather to cars trying to run him off the road to support-car troubles to two fractured ankles (obviously not compound fractures) to loneliness and depression. Yet through it all, he held tenaciously onto his vision to help children and consequently, made it to his destination, Centennial Park, in Atlanta and the home and start of the 1996 Summer Olympics.

Thanks to his resolve, he now inspires young and old with motivational talks on his 2,000-mile odyssey, perseverance, goal setting, and his tale of success. Terry went on to be president of Ed View, Inc., a successful internet company; serve on a White House panel to keep kids safe; and take a position with Hyperport International (a theme park for the mind).

If Terry, a 56-year-old raising teenagers by himself, with little running experience, can run the equivalent of 75 marathons in 75 days, then WE CAN train to participate in a local walkathon to raise money for a worthy cause or train for a Team Diabetes Marathon (see www.diabetes.org /teamdiabetes for details) or we can ....

How You Gonna Keep Him Down On The Farm?
Why would one leave the idyllic life of a sheep farmer in Tussock Creek, New Zealand to travel to a crowded, noisy, pollution-friendly city across the world? Despite all the work on a farm (or maybe because of it) what with 3,000 sheep to care for, big ewes to shear, cows to milk, eggs to gather, **Derek Turnbull** finds time to travel to the far corners of the world to compete as a world-class runner. He does it for the contrast; to enjoy the carnival atmosphere of competitions; and to have the fun of travel.

Despite the fact that he considers running just a hobby, claims he doesn't train (just runs when and where he feels like it), and takes the winters off from running, he continued year after year to set age-group world records in everything from 800-meter "dashes" to marathons.

Here's the kicker! In 1987 he decided to be the first 60-year-old to break 2 hours and 40 minutes in a marathon, which he did at Adelaide with a 2:38:46. What is most significant to our topic of getting fitter after 50 is that after 48 years of running it was his personal best ever in the marathon. My calculations say that he ran just over 6 minutes per mile. Considering that most men could never run a single mile that fast at any age, and that the top marathoners of the day were running just over 5 minutes a mile, this is amazing! It shows that we really can get better with age.

Derek had been running since age 13 and claimed that he was not especially talented. He said that he just hadn't slowed down. According to author, Roger Robinson, Derek's 800 meter/half mile times stayed at 2 minutes and 6 seconds from age 18, in 1945, to age 58 in 1985; at age 70 it was still under 2:30.

To what can we attribute this staying power through the years? I would say that the daily exercise and the hard work of running a farm prepared him to endure the pain of world-elite championship-level long distance running. Also, listening to his body (i.e., running when he felt like it — when he was inspired to drop everything and take a run) contributed to his mastery and kept him fresh. Add to this an iron will, a competitor's heart, and a love for running/racing and you have the secrets to his improving with age as an elite-level international competitor.

Remember, the average person, such as you and I, does not need to endure painful workouts (maybe a little discomfort as we challenge ourselves to reach beyond our current comfort zone, but not pain) to improve our fitness because the less fit one is, the less work it takes to get better. At Derek's level of competition, pain is a given. For most of us, suffering through workouts is not only unnecessary, but counter-productive to our getting fitter.

If Derek can improve with age at an elite level and maintain such high fitness standards, maybe we can improve our fitness and health by increasing the distance of our walks, the number of push-ups or crunches we can complete in 1 minute, or setting personal bests for the mile run. Maybe we would even enjoy competing in our age-group in some local races.

Late Bloomers Are Better Than No Bloomers At All

It's not unusual for women to dedicate their lives to raising their children and supporting their husbands in their endeavers (Lord knows they need it). **Lois Lindsay** was such a woman, a stay-at-home mom who put all her energies into doing for her family, in her case three wonderful children and a loving husband.

At 42, having supported her husband and son from the sidelines at their cycling competitions, Lois decided to try biking herself. She thought it might be fun and something she could do *with* her family as opposed to just doing *for* them all the time. So she borrowed a ladies bike and set off on an inaugural 7-mile jaunt. This little ride left her totally exhausted — physically wiped out. She had discovered that she had no endurance. Yet, despite the pain and utter fatigue, she found it exhilerating, too.

Using the discipline she had acquired growing up on a farm, Lois decided to keep at it so that she could ride with her family. At first she couldn't keep up at all and so she increased her training, adding 1 mile runs to build her endurance. Due to her increased training, finally she could ride comfortably with her husband and son.

From there she was inspired to try a 100-mile ride. Along the way, she discovered a competitive spirit she didn't know she had; growing up in the country, she wasn't exposed to any sports, just farming. She didn't even own a bike as a kid. This desire to bike race and compete appeared to come out of nowhere; as a child she had wanted to be an artist and even majored in art in college.

Through much practice, the support of her family, and learning the tricks of the trade through a biking club she joined, Lois got better and better to the point of qualifying for the Nationals at age 44. At the national competition she felt completely intimidated by the other highly-trained, top riders in the country.

Instead of quiting, she entered every local race she could find, gaining more and more experience and skill. In 1986, at age 51, Lois made a major breakthrough, setting a national record in her age group, in the 40K (about 25 miles) time trial. She has since earned three more national titles and at age 65 was still getting better.

Lois never dreamed that biking, or any sport for that matter, would change her life so dramatically. Remember, she had just wanted to have some fun doing something (anything) she could do *with* her family. Through her "late"-in-life discovery of cycling competition, Lois has been able to travel the world, receive her share of accolades, and stay in incredible shape while "eating anything I want to."

Lois wasn't born an athlete. She had no sports role models growing up. She could have been and stayed a couch potato all her life. Instead she became a champion athlete and a fitness role model for us. Lois has shown us that we can become an athlete at any stage of our life. If Lois can do it , then maybe we can take up ice skating, rock climbing, or ... *AND become really good at it* — maybe even enjoy competing for ribbons and trophies — even at our age!

Asthma Attacks Disappear With Exercise

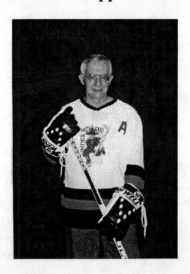

Hockey player/runner, **Kenneth "Ice" Morrison,** had recently turned 60 when we sat down at our respective computers to do this E-Interview. It has been pieced together from two separate interviews, several months apart.

FA50: Do you consider yourself fitter than you were as a younger adult and/or fitter than the average 30 or 40-year-old? If so, what is your criterion for thinking thusly?

Ken: I am in much better physical shape than I was up to the age of 35. I was always active, but suffered from asthma and used that as an excuse not to really be that active. Once I started, and continued, with a good physical regimen, the asthma slowly disappeared. The criteria for my better physical shape are: I can now accomplish physical exercise, whether it be sport, yard work, housework, etc. — do it longer, enjoy it, and feel good afterwards.

FA50: Could you elaborate on the asthma disappearing?

Ken: I started running in 1975 as cross training for my hockey. As I got more involved in running (i.e., building up the miles, running longer races), I noticed that the frequency of my "shortness of breath" attacks dropped off significantly. I used OTC relief for the attacks and found that the bottles were expiring before I used them up! I always kept an inhaler with my running and hockey gear, but as time went on, the need [for it] grew less and less. In fact, about the only time I had need for the inhaler was during the Spring allergy seasons. After a long inactive period due to surgery, I saw a slight increase in the the usage of the inhaler. Of course, right now is peak allergy season, so I suspect that is a contributor. I am now back to a running/hockey program and expect a decrease once again.

FA50: Tell us more about your exercise/sports regimen (please!).

Ken: Around age 35 to 36 I started playing ice hockey again (I had played as a child). I also started running as a cross-training exercise, and running became the dominant physical activity until 55 when I went back to hockey (roller-blade type in an over-30 league: held my own with the younger crowd!).

FA50: Any specific signs that you are in better shape now beyond what you have already told us?

Ken: Can't really say right now, as I have just fully recovered from hernia surgery. I am back full time at hockey and I have started my running program, so I should be back in shape for the Corporate Track and Field Championships in

July. I think I am [in] fairly fit shape as I can keep up with people half my age in hockey — the key is pacing. I know I can't match them step-for-step continuously — but if I spend two minutes on and two off, I can keep up. Of course "old age and treachery will overcome youth and enthusiasm" most of the time!! And, I have been asked back for the Fall season, as well as being invited to play in another league! I think one of the key indicators of fitness (at least for me) is sleep. I have no trouble going to sleep, and I sleep deeply and wake up refreshed. I average 6 hours a night - more and I tend to feel a bit sluggish the next day.

FA50: To what do you attribute your fitness — your ability to play hockey at age 60, etc.?

Ken: Establishing and staying with somewhat of a regimen of exercise. Eliminating excuses for not exercising. Meeting a variety of people, and establishing new friendships. And, I think when you are physically fit, the mental stresses are easier to cope with.

FA50: What is your diet like?

Ken: Ordinary diet — eat just about anything. I Try to keep the red meat intake low because my digestive system seems to work better when I do. What do I eat? The four basic food groups: Pasta, beer, scotch, and chocolate!! Seriously, just about anything — I try to limit the amount per serving — I feel overeating is where the weight comes from. What don't I eat? Eggplant!

FA50: Do you take any supplements, such as vitamins, protein powders, etc.?

Ken: Yes: 400 IU vitamin E; 500 mg Vitamin C complex; 500 mg L-Lysine [an amino acid]; 30 mg zinc; "OneSource" multi-vitamin; Trader Joe's Antioxidant and Xioa Yao Wan. If I have an evening hockey game, I take a multi-vitamin, antioxidant, and a "C" about two hours before the game — don't know if it does any good, but I feel I have an increase in energy above what I have when I don't take them.

FA50: And finally, Ken, what advice would you give to a Senior thinking about starting an exercise program?

Ken: Two answers here: one for those who have exercised before and one for those who have not.

Have not exercised before:
- Get a physical
- Do some research into the activity you are interested in
- Set realistic goals
- Obtain proper equipment
- Find a group with like interests and work with them
- Listen to your body!
- Don't overdo a workout because you are feeling great
- Rest
- Maintain a good diet
- Have patience — you won't get fit overnight
- Don't worry about your appearance

Have exercised before:
- All the above — plus
- You are not as fast or as agile as you were when you were younger — remember that!
- Have more patience — you can't get back into shape as fast as you used to

Hope this helps some.

FA50: It does and it will. Good advice — thanks!

A Locomotive With Legs

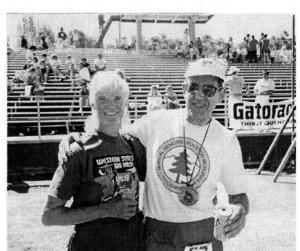

Dick Collins with his best friend and training partner, Ruth Anderson

At age 41, in 1975, a doctor told **Dick Collins,** a more than 60-pounds overweight smoker, that he had better make some lifestyle changes or else. So Dick changed his diet, quit smoking (eventually), and took up running — boy, did he ever take up running! In the next 21 or so years, he completed 1,000 races with more than 250 of them at least 30 miles or more.

By 1986 he had run 100 ultra-marathons *AND finished every one of them.* When Dick set out to do something, he did it! He became so accomplished that in July of 1984, having already turned 51, he won the Gator 24-Hour Race by self-propelling himself 116 miles. The next year he set an American record for 52-year-olds, in a Santa Rosa 24-hour race, with a run of 111.5 miles. *Dick went on to run a staggering 800-plus consecutive foot-races without ever dropping out of one!*

You are probably thinking that he was a born runner and that at 41 his runner's body was just hidden under a facade of flab and tar-filled lungs, that unlike us, he was genetically predisposed to be a natural at running. However, this was not the case. He more resembled a wrestler than a long-distance runner as he competed in the ultras carrying a solid 180 pounds on his 5-foot-10-inch frame — not exactly the lithe, streamline, all-legs physique of the typical champion long-distance runner. Like a locomotive, he chugged along — mile after mile of determined resolve. He was like the Little Engine That Could — only larger.

You would think that with all that fresh air and exercise (not to mention his improved diet and smoke-free lungs) he would live forever or least into "old age," but alas, Dick died of a heart attack at age 63. Did he die by pushing too hard during a grueling race? No, he passed on while watching TV.

What can we learn from Dick? One thing is that we can make ourselves — transform ourselves — into a top caliber athlete, musician, or whatever even if our body and/or mind is not a perfect match for the skill. We can see clearly that we can change dramatically — even after age 40. Finally, the traits that made Dick so successful were his determination, perseverance, and focus. He must have pushed himself through Hell to complete some of those ultra-long races. He undoubtedly ignored or subordinated some serious, major pain signals/warning signs from his body to complete more than 800-straight *long distance and ultra-long distance races.* Maybe, just maybe, the traits that made him a champion, that allowed him to show us just how much more we are capable of than we tend to believe, at 63, did him in.

One can over-train, get too much exercise, and race too hard, too often. A fit body is not always a healthy body; witness the champion athletes who seem to have all-too-frequent bouts with sickness and injuries. We need to listen to what our body tells us and balance our periods of exertion with sufficient rest. Then again, maybe Dick's family history of heart trouble just caught up with him.

The quality of one's life is what is important, not the length; sooner or later we will all be gone. Dick was adored in the ultra-running community. His fellow runners say he was always there to help. When he wasn't leading by example — running in races — he was "running" races —volunteering to do whatever needed to be done to make a race successful. He was legendary for dropping whatever he was doing to answer the questions of neophytes and generously share his knowledge and wisdom. Ruth Anderson says it best, "Of course he was 'my best friend,' but such a friend to others ... perhaps the most 'encouraging' and supporting of runners of every age and level."

If Dick could finish race after race, no matter how many miles were involved, then WE CAN complete 30 minutes of exercise on a regular basis. Thus we will be able to enjoy the activities that we love and make the most of each day of our earthly sojourn, whether we live a long or short life.

Too Busy To Exercise, ...

Like **Dr. Wayne Dyer**, we may be so busy with all our family obligations that we have little time to exercise. For Dr. Dyer it's a wife and eight children to love, support, chaffeur, and cheer (school plays, sporting events, graduations, ...). Of course work (i.e., a career) tends to put the kibosh on a convenient workout schedule or any consistent fitness program at all. In Dr. Dyer's case that includes writing 14 books (with writing deadlines) and being a guest on over 5,200 TV and radio shows over a 25-year span (the way I figure it, that's over 200 interviews per year, not counting print). Being one of the most sought-after speakers in the country, it also means constant air travel with its frustrating, schedule-juggling delays and cancellations. So you see, one couldn't expect Dr. Dyer to get in his workouts on a regular basis — just as we can't with our hectic, modern-day, mind-boggling schedules.

But wait! Stop the presses! Dr. Dyer does manage, somehow, to work out consistently. How consistently? According to WayneDyer.com, "Dr. Dyer includes among his most satisfying accomplishments the fact that he has run a minimum of eight miles a day every day since 1976." As of this writing, that is about 25 years without missing a daily run. Think about it. No matter what the deadlines, what the travel contingencies, what the children were up to, what the heck — he found time to take care of himself. Lest you think that Dr. Dyer has the exclusive bragging rights, there are dozens of such "streak runners," as they are called, and even a web site devoted to them. For example, as of 1999, Bob Ray, 61, of Baltimore, MD, had run every day since 1967 and Walter Byerly, 68, of Dallas TX had run a consecutive string dating back to 1974 (to name 2 who have surpassed Dr. Dyer).

What Dr. Dyer did was put himself first because he knew that he wasn't much good to his family, or readers/"followers," if he was too sick or tired or worse, too dead, to support, love, and assist them. Therefore, most mornings he got up at 4:45 AM and ran 12 to 15 miles miles. He is now (as of 2001) 61 and as far as I know still going strong; so I guess the knee and hip joints can take a lot more pounding than we tend to think. Also, he walks to the store instead of driving, when practical, and negotiates flights of stairs instead of taking the elevator. In addition he meditates for about 20 minutes at the beginning and end of each day (exercise for the soul).

Three things are evident from this:
1. *Mrs.* Dyer must be a Saint!
2. Exercise doesn't prevent baldness (if you've ever seen Wayne you know what I mean)
3. Excuses not to exercise, or otherwise take care of ourselves, are just that.

If Wayne Dyer can find the time to work out and meditate on a daily basis, then maybe we can (okay, okay, maybe not 15 miles, but...) We can feel good about making this commitment because we *know* that one of the best things we can do for our family is to take care of ourself so that we'll be around for a long, long time to support them, encourage them, love them and be loved by them!

Postscript — *Just before going to press I learned that Dr. Dyer had recently suffered a heart attack. Dr. Dyer said it was due to a genetic condition and that it has been fixed and he is back to his running. What can we glean from Dr. Dyer's misfortune?*

1. *Exercise, in this case running, is not a guarantee of wellness; it merely greatly increases our odds of getting fit and staying well — when it is done intelligently.*
2. *There are more factors that support our well-being than just getting the exercise we need and we can overdo a good thing!*
3. *In order to continue a "streak of running," one must run on some days when the body would be better served by rest due to a fever, a twisted ankle that needs time to heal, or a host of other possible maladies. In order to keep his streak alive, one has to ignore these signals or requests from the body for time off. This ability and desire to run despite pain or discomfort can lead to disregarding signs of more serious conditions until it is "too late."*
4. *Dr. Dyer had just completed his latest book, "There's a Spiritual Solution To Every Problem"— makes one think, doesn't it?*

Bernie Siegel, MD

Dr. Bernie Siegel is a surgeon turned mind-body expert, lecturing extensively on the subject. He has also penned two best-selling books, *Love, Medicine And Miracles* and *How To Live Between Office Visits*. Despite or because of these time-consuming activities and duties at his Mind-Body Wellness Center (depending on your point of view), he runs — a lot. Every morning he goes for a run of at least an hour; giving him plenty of time for introspection and to listen to his "inner voice." In his sixty-fourth year he ran The New York City Marathon for the sixth time. As with Dr. Dyer, he also finds time to meditate.

Concerning his running, in a 1997 interview with Peter Barry Chowka, he said, "Everyone can be like me. Some of it is me taking care of me ..." I believe he would tell you that he doesn't do this so as not to die, but rather to maximize his life experience. His diet is not extreme or rigid, and even with all the running (actually, partly because of it) he enjoys life. In the aforementioned interview, he said that we could have healthy adults who, when they get tired of living, die easily and we could also have healthy individuals who don't cost a lot.

Long-term care costs in America today can easily be 40-to $100,000 per year, and are rising faster than inflation. Individuals who didn't bother to take care of themselves in their middle years often become frail, sickly aged ones who unmercifully *hang on* for a decade or more.

Would you agree that we don't want to saddle our family and country with this staggering emotional and financial price tag? If you do, then we, like Dr. Siegel, must take care of ourselves. When we put our own health and well-being first, everyone wins!

Ironmen All

Those of you who have at some time caught ABC Sports' annual coverage of the Hawaiian Ironman Triathlon know that this is a brutal test of one's endurance and physical fitness. This 3-part race is definitely not for old geezers, in that it starts with a 2.4-mile ocean swim; continues without a break (other than a quick costume change) with a 112-mile bike race; and concludes with a mere 26-mile marathon run. Wooh! I get tired just describing it. Yet, some individuals well past 50 have the audacity to compete and do well, even though they should be slowing down and taking it easy as they get ready to retire, hang around the house, get underfoot, and drive their mates crazy (not to mention making their reservations for the old folks' home).

Let's take a look at what we "oldsters" can accomplish when we put our mind (and body) to it.

Robert McKeague, at age 57, went on a family ski trip. After a single day on the slopes, he was so sore and exhausted that he had to spend the whole next day in bed recuperating. This was a wake-up call for him, letting him know that he was really out of shape. Well, that was 18 years ago, and he has made some changes. For example, in 1997 he competed in the Hawaiian Ironman Triathlon and finished first in the 70-to-74 age group with an impressive time of 14 hours and 50 minutes. One could safely assume that he is in better shape now than when he was much younger AND more fit than 99.9 percent of our 20-and 30-somethings.

Another mature triathlete is **Bob Scott.** Working 50 hours a week as a senior engineer and spending time with his family (wife and 2 sons), one might think that Bob wouldn't have time to train 25-27 hours per week, but he does. The result — Hawaiian Ironman successes: 1997 - 14:22:03; 1999 - 13:37:51; AND, 2000 - 13:13:32. As you can clearly see, his times are getting better with age, as attested to by the fact that his 2000 race at age 70 is his best ever.

If you are thinking that it's easy for men (with their wives taking care of family matters and feeding them, etc.) to fit triathlons, with all their prerequisite training, into their schedules, but that women, especially working mothers, could never find the time or energy to run triathlons, then meet **Ethel Autorino**. Ethel managed to raise four children, work a full-time job, and still have time to train as a triathlete, 20 to 25 hours each week. How'd she do it? She would run at 5 AM, come home, get her kids off to school, and then head off for a full-day's work. She also managed to squeeze in training runs during lunch breaks and on weekends.

Ethel competed in her first triathlon at age 55. But first she had to buy a bike, since she hadn't owned or ridden one since she was a little girl. She went on to a 13:23 in the Hawaiian Ironman at age 56. Since then she's completed the Ironman in 1990 at age 60; in 1995 at 65; and in 2000 at 70-years-*young.* AND, her 2000 time was about 14 minutes faster than her 1995 score even though her foot was so swollen just two days before the race that she couldn't even walk. Now Ethel is going to take some time off for a leisurely sight-seeing trip across the contiguous United States with her biking club — a nice, easy 3,200-mile bike ride.

During his thirties and forties, physical fitness was not part of **Roger Brockenbrough's** active vocabulary, as he was busy putting bread on the table and helping his wife raise their four children. Then in 1985, at age 51, after watching his son compete in races, he decided to get back in shape himself. He had done an occasional run or swim, but nothing that could be mistaken for training. Roger decided to try a triathlon (a smaller version — *not* the Ironman size) and won a trophy and that's all it took; he was off and running — and biking — and swimming.

Roger trains hard: swimming 7,000-8,000 yards; biking 100 miles; and running 20 miles weekly. When there is a competition coming up he ups it to 10-12,000 yards of swimming, 150 miles biking, and 25-30 miles of running. Living in Pittsburgh, Pennsylvania, in the winter he sometimes has to substitute stair climbing at the University of Pennsylvania: 36 flights in 6.5 to 7 minutes; walk back down; and repeat 5 more times. It's paid off with his winning the 65 - 69 age-group in the 2000 Hawaiian Ironman with a 14:08:59.

Since **Richard Clark** turned 60, he's been practically nothing but gold. Among his trophies is first place at the 2000 World Long Distance Triathlon Championships in Nice (probably in Italy). Also, Triathlon Magazine named him the 2000 Male Amateur Triathlete of the Year — beating, I might add, *all* the fantastic 20, 30 and 40-year-old triathletes. That's quite an accomplishment for someone on the back nine of life and who didn't enter his first triathlon until 1989, when he was already 51. To get these accolades, Richard swims 8 miles, bikes 200-plus miles, and runs 40 miles each week using a cross-training approach (i.e., running one day, biking another day, etc.). Does that sound like the training schedule of an old codger? I think not!

Finally, there is **Sister Madonna Buder**, a nun, who heard a seminar about the benefits of running in 1978 and decided to try it. Training for her first race, an 8.2-miler, she suffered through every ache and pain known to man (or woman), except for childbirth. A couple of years later, at age 52, she had worked her way up to her first marathon. Now in her seventies, she has completed a stagering 200-plus triathlons, including 13 Hawaiian Ironmans — setting records in two age divisions along the way. But it hasn't always been easy, as

Sister Madonna has suffered *and overcome* a broken hip, fractured elbow and jaw and broken ribs along the way.

What motivates these seniors to take on such an arduous, physically challenging, seemingly impossible undertaking? Aren't we supposed to take it easy in our reclining years? What drives them is the camaraderie, accolades, sense of accomplishment, direction, and opportunity to be good role models for the rest of us, young and old. They literally jump at the chance to show us, and themselves, the untapped potential we have that knows no age boundaries. They thrive on extending and expanding the boundaries, and knocking down the barriers, of our self-imposed, illusionary limits built on the false belief that aging means a steady decline to the grave. Or as Captain Kirk might say, "They revel in going where no man has gone before!"

If Robert, Bob, Ethel, Roger, Richard and Sister Madonna can train and race this hard and live such rich and rewarding lives, then we can look forward to not just surviving through our later years, but actually thriving — if we make our well-being our top priority.

She's Got Game

Team captain for the Loiusiana 50-plus Hi-Tops Tigerettes basketball team is **Mavis Albin**, 64. When Mavis started playing again in her early fifties (she loved hoops in high school), she was "… exhausted after two minutes" because she hadn't exercised regularly in years. Now she has the energy and stamina to run the court for whole ball games without even so much as a nap at halftime. Mavis really is fitter after 50!

Since 1993, Albin and her six teammates have won Gold Medals three times at the Senior Olympics and are 62 and 2 while barnstorming the country playing other "seasoned" basketball teams.

If Mavis can so successfully and wholeheartedly take up the sport she loved as a youngster, then maybe we can put some joy and excitement back in our life by lacing up our sneakers or sharpening our ice skates, or … and revisiting our sports passions from years gone by.

It's the Little Things That Count

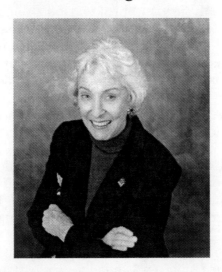

In **Janet Baker-Murray's** home you won't find a trophy case to attest to her athletic prowess. There are no world or national records for races won, not even regional or local ones, although she has run the Bay to Breakers 10K in San Francisco. So why is Janet's story in this chapter with all the sports champions? She's here for you to meet because not all of us can be athletic or fitness champions, nor do we all want to be; and after all, it's the little things that make life enjoyable.

We refer to little things such as younger men asking the 65-year-old mother of 6 if she is an athlete. This definitely strokes one's ego — I know it would mine. Little things such as other women, her competitors in the game of life, asking silently *and* aloud how she stays so young — looks so much younger than her chronological age. Since men tend to turn up their toes years before women do, this can come in handy with the inevitable dearth of available mature men in case your soul mate #1 takes a premature dirt nap. And little things, such as teaching piano to elite young-adult pianists preparing for competitions, such as the Van Cliburn Competition Adjudication. Janet's abundance of energy allows her to instruct these developing piano virtuosos (and even take them to perform in Europe — Edinburgh, London, Paris, ... — as the Concert Masters) with no plans for retirement in the forseeable future despite nearing "retirement age." She also has the stamina to tutor these pianists in the evening with the resultant frequent midnight bedtime (meanwhile I'm falling asleep at the keyboard in the middle of the afternoon as I write this — abruptly waking to see two lines of nothing but "L's" as my finger rested on that key as I took a mini-slumber AND grateful that I didn't create *pages of "L's"*).

To reap these fitness benefits, Janet, a smoker for 23 years and now smoke free for a similar length of time, exercises for an hour, five times per week. This has included running, step-aerobics, body sculpting, stretching/flexibility exercises, balance training, light weight lifting, and hiking (in the Swiss Alps this past year). And, although she has only been in a gym twice, Janet has also been a swimmer and a golfer.

Janet's diet of mostly fruits, vegetables, whole multi-grains, seeds, and nuts helps her maintain her amazing youthful appearance and vigor; as does staying away from icky-sweet foods (most of the time) and forsaking sodas.

Janet is a true ambassador for fitness after 50. Her lifestyle is a wonderful model for all of us. If Janet can exude fitness and vibrancy wherever she goes and whatever she's doing, then so can we. We want to be a role model for young and old and an ambassador for fitness and radiant well-being, too, and so we are going to commit to _____.

Getting Faster All the Time

It's not unusual for an individual who's been relatively sedentary for years or even decades to take up a sport, such as running, biking or even golf and realistically look forward to 10 or 15 years of improving scores — an ever upgrading of his skill level. What is quite uncommon is for an elite athlete over the age of 40 to better his best scores from his youth, but this is exactly what **Rich Abrahams**, 53, has done.

Rich is the first over-50 athlete to break 50 seconds in a 100-yard freestyle swimming race. His 48.8 seconds for the 100 would make many elite college swimmers envious. This score is more than a full second faster (in a sport where hundredths of a second is often all that separates first place from second and third place) than he could swim it 6 years earlier, at age 47. His 50-free time is actually *faster* than it was when he was in college, some 30 years earlier.

31

To put his 100-free score in perspective, let's compare it with Olympic Games' times. First, since they swim meter distances (not yards) in the Olympics, we've done some math and found that a 48.8 100-yard time converts to about a 52.8 100-meter score. This having been done, we find that this 53-year-old would have just missed the qualifying time for the 2000 Sydney Olympic Games by about two-tenths of a second; and his time is just 1.2 seconds slower than Mark Spitz' Gold Medal swim at the 1972 Games. Not bad for an "old-timer"!

How does Rich do it? He trains hard, putting in his laps similar to the training the Olympians endure. He also lifts weights diligently. This helps account for the fact that he can jump up from a standing-still position and grab a standard, 10-foot-high basketball rim and hang on it (something only a rare few 20-year-old elite athletes can do).

At 53, Rich is fully intending and believing that he can get faster. He knows there are little things he can improve to get even faster, such as a quicker start or perhaps increasing his shoulder flexibility so he can increase his reach on each stroke.

If Rich at his elite level can continue to get faster, then maybe we can take up a sport with similar prospects of getting better and better for years to come. By talking to experienced competitors, reading books by experts, joining a club/group and training intelligently WE CAN make this dream a reality; we can enjoy and compete in the sport of our choice successfully no matter what our chronological age.

The Great Six-Day Races

The great 6-day races date back to the 1870's when they were called Pedestrianism and the best American pedestrians were Edward Payson Weston and Daniel O'Leary. In 1884 one of the best pedestrian races ever was between Brit, Charles Rowell and Irishman, Patrick Fitzgerald and 11 other racers. Six-day mania swept the US as 10,000 spectators crowded into Madison Square Garden for the big event. To make an amazing, suspenseful story short, in a seesaw race, Fitzgerald won with 610 miles covered to Rowell's 602.

But, that was then and this is now (and neither Rowell nor Fitzgerald was 50-plus), so what does all this have to do with being fitter after 50? Just this. In May of 1998, on Ward's Island, New York, just across the river from Manhattan, the Sri

Chinmoy Six-Day Races were held. Despite rain falling during almost the entire race, 5 inches in all, the runners were able to somehow negotiate the huge puddles and gobs of mud as they circled the one-mile loop time after time.

Istvan Sipos, 38, of Szeged, Hungary won by covering 670 miles over the 6 days of competition, but he had to withstand a blistering "eleventh-hour" challenge from **Georgs Jermolajevs** of Riga, Latvia, who in his final charge made up 17 miles in the last 8 hours, only to lose by a single mile - 669 to 670. Here's the kicker, the significant part for us — Jermolajevs was *55-years-old!*

Likewise, in the women's division of the 6-day event, it's not the winner that we are so interested in, one Dipali Cunningham, 38, of Melbourne, Australia, with a world road best (and callous forming) 504 miles. What is striking, from our point of view, is that second place again goes to a 50-plus runner. In this case, Brit, **Pippa Davis**, 51, was runner-up with 414 miles.

If the over-50 crowd can represent themselves this well in these grueling ultra-endurance races, then maybe we can regain an energy level, a degree of stamina, that will allow us to work all day and still have boundless energy to enjoy our evenings, instead of crashing on the couch, falling into bed only to wake up the next morning tired and with the uninspiring prospect of having to do it all over again.

Stair Masters

What would possess someone to forsake a perfectly good elevator, one of modern man's technological marvels, to take the arduous climb up the steps of a sky-scraper? What that something is, is a stair-climbing competition, a race up *several* flights of stairs.

Remember the last time you sprinted up a couple of flights of stairs (or should we say "survived" two flights) and how breathless you were when you got to the top? Now imagine hundreds of eager stair racers crowded together at the foot of the steps to some high-rise building, jostling for position. Can you see them, as the starter's pistol goes off, elbowing each other out of the way and climbing over each other, like Archie Bunker and Meathead trying to get through a small doorway at the same time?

Actually, you can forget that image because climbers take off at 10-second intervals in a *staggered* start sequence; and stagger is just what most of us would be doing after the first dozen or so flights.

Stair-climbing competitions started in the mid-1970s and now include climbs up the Hancock Center in Chicago, the Los Angeles Library Tower, the Nation's Bank Tower in Dallas, and New York City's Empire State Building among others.

We'll start with one of Los Angeles' recent races up the 75-story Library Tower and see how some Master athletes fared. On the men's side, winning his age division was a 65-year-old electrical engineer from Indianapolis, Indiana, **Steve Wilson**. Steve's award-winning time was 14 minutes and 37 seconds. That's less than 11 seconds per flight for 75 flights; not much time to stop and catch one's breath, and not bad for someone of "retirement age." It was Steve's fifteenth year as a stair-climbing competitor. Representing the Masters women was **Joanne Keaton**, 67, another Hoosier (and I thought Indiana was flat like most of the midwest), with an age-group win of 18:19 — less than 15 seconds per floor — very impressive indeed!

The Hustle Up the Hancock is a 94-floor challenge. It consists of a 1,000 foot vertical climb up 1,632 stair steps to raise money for the American Lung Association. In 2001 there were over 400 competitors with a good sprinkling of 50-plusers. First among the senior women, again, was Joanne Keaton with a time of 19:51; leading the men in his age group was **Paul Levy**, 64, of Glencoe, Illinois, in 16:09. By comparison, the overall women's winner turned in a time of 14:15; the men's champion scored a lightening quick 11:31. So you can see that Joanne and Paul represented us, the older crowd, admirably.

The oldest finisher ever in the Empire State Building Run Up was **Chico Simone** who was 89, in 2001, when he scaled this American treasure like King Kong before him. Runner's World magazine reported him as saying, "I just want to be an example to everyone. Eighty-nine is an age you should look forward to."

We may or may not be turned on by the prospect of racing up 80 or 90 flights of steps, but we all can take the stairs in lieu of the elevator (or escalator) for an occasional or regular workout; maybe we can make it a regular part of our everyday life.

A recent study at the University of Ulster, in Northern Ireland, cited the benefits of stair climbing. They took 12 healthy, but sedentary college-age women, put them on a stair-climbing regimen, and compared them with a control group that did no stair climbing. They had the young ladies ascend six flights of steps, starting with just one flight at first and gradually working up to the six flights per day. Each flight consisted of 199 steps and took approximately 2 minutes and 15 seconds to ascend. Scaling the whole six flights took just thirteen and a half minutes a day. For this small investment of time, when compared to the non-exercising control group, their heart rates were lower, they used oxygen more efficiently, and their ratio of HDL "good" cholesterol to total cholesterol was 20% better.

Any strenuous activity could probably produce similar results, but stair climbing is nice because one can easily make it a part of his/her day by simply substituting the stairs for the elevator (if one works in a high-rise building, that is) with no change of clothes, no trips to the gym, or other inconveniences necessary. As an added bonus, you may even save time and aggravation by avoiding long waits for the elevator, as well as escaping being crammed together like sardines (with imperfect strangers) for the often uncomfortable ride. Furthermore, walking up and down stairs can improve posture, help prevent osteoporosis, and strengthen and sculpt the lower body.

If Steven, Joanne, Paul, and Chico can bound up 75 to 96 flights, then maybe we can make a few stair climbs or other vigorous activity, such as high-speed "power" cleaning, a regular part of our hectic schedule.

The Norm Green Interview

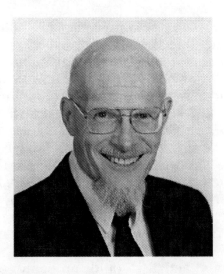

Norm Green is an ardent ambassador of competitive running, Masters running and fitness in general and as such has held several administrative positions on the USATF (USA Track & Field) and WAVA (World Association of Veteran Athletes — in 2001 renamed, World Masters Athletics, WMA). Norm has much to teach us about being fitter after 50. Although he was a good runner in his youth, he didn't start running again until his late thirties, and didn't return to the sport (i.e., running competitively) until his late 40s; and according to author, Roger Robinson, in a *Marathon and Beyond* magazine article, "Norm achieved the rare satisfaction of recording his set of lifetime personal records in 1983-84 when he was over 51." This was rare because he was able to surpass his times from when he was a track star at Piedmont High. On the other hand, it is not unusual for those of us who have never excelled at a particular sport to take up that activity later in life and become extremely proficient at it or much better than we ever were in our earlier days, and to set new personal bests over a span of years. And now Norm's interview:

FA50: Norm, thank you for the privilege of interviewing you. First, what would you like to tell our readers about becoming fitter after 50?

36

Norm: Get clearance from an MD/OD before you start an exercise regimen. It is never too late to start. Although exercise may not prolong your life, it will, without question, improve your quality of life.

FA50: What kind of shape were you in before you started running again?

Norm: After I stopped running in 1952 (age 20), I did NO exercise until challenged in 1968 by the Elmhurst (IL) Recreation Department to join a "joggers' club." At first I could not run around a city block without stopping to walk and recover my breath. Three years later I was running 50-70 miles a week.

FA50: To what do you attribute your world and national record-setting success in your fifties?

Norm: Primarily a genetic gift, enhanced by a significant level of aerobic exercise (walking, running, cycling) from age 9 through 20. That foundation was coupled with forced nutritional benefits of the Depression and World War II food rationing. I lived in California and had the advantage of home-grown fruits and vegetables and never acquired a taste for "junk food."

FA50: Can individuals 50 and older become fitter than most 20-and-30-year-olds?

Norm: Any individual who is motivated to improve her/his quality of life at any age in the lifespan can become fitter than the average 20 to 30-year-old. Fitness requires a mindset that the early aches and pains accompanying exercises are worth enduring for the sake of what lies on the other side.

FA50: What benefits did you accrue from returning to competitive running in your your forties, fifties and sixties?

Norm: In the early years of my racing career (1981-1995) I reduced my weight 20 pounds, achieving a "look of fitness" that was the envy of friends and acquaintances. Road racing enabled my wife and me to travel to competitions in France, Finland, Belgium, England, Israel, Australia, Korea, South Africa, Trinidad, Mexico, Barbados, and Canada. I literally do have friends, made from these contacts, all over the world. My resting heart rate was lowered to 36-40 bpm. Healthwise, for much of that career I was able to withstand extremely high work stress without ill effect. However, by 1992 the accumulated stress of my work and other life involvements overcame the running-related benefits leading to three serious illnesses (pneumonia, prostatitis, Hashimoto's thyroiditis) across the year and ultimately to my decison to take early retirement in 1995 from my denominational position of 33 years.

The diagnosis of prostate cancer in the fall of 1995 was followed by surgery in June, 1996. I lost 18 months of training and racing throughout the process and have never recovered my speed or stamina since that layoff. I am now a recreational runner rather than the elite Masters runner I was before 1993.

FA50: Tell us about your racing career, both as a high school runner and then as a Masters runner.

Norm: In high school I ran the mile as a junior and senior. Across those 2 years I was undefeated in the mile run throughout the dual meet season and through the Association and Regional meets in Northern California (I attended Piedmont High School, Piedmont, CA). Although I placed poorly in the state meet, I have always prized the accomplishment of those two spring seasons as an enhancement of my self-esteem and peer recognition. My distance running in those days was primarily multitudes of laps on the track. Other track athletes would "relay" me, while I maintained a steady pace lap after lap. I was given the nickname "the machine" by my peers.

In my first major Masters national championship (May, 1983), I was running with the lead pack for the first two laps of the Haines Point course in Washington, DC. The race was the National Masters 20k [12.4 miles]. As we began the third lap only one other runner, who happened to be 40 to my age of 50, went with me as I slightly increased the pace. By the fourth lap I was running alone, with all the 40-year-olds convinced I would come back to them. However, I was running for the national record and easily won the race (1:05:50). That victory established my national reputation and proved to be the first of ultimately 8 OVERALL masters national championships won after the age of 50 (the last in 1987 at the age of 55). No other Masters road racer over the age of 50 has won an overall national championship, while I did it 8 times. I really believe that is a record that will never be broken.

FA50: My math says that your 20k (1:05:50) was about a 5 minute and 20 second per mile pace; AND 8 Masters national championships in your fifties while competing with 40-year-olds (not to mention your amazing 2:27:42 Twin Cities Marathon at age 55) — Wow! What was your training like to do that?

Norm: During my heyday (1982-1992) my weekly average was between 50 and 60 miles. In most of those years I was running 7 days per week, interspersing long and short days (3 miles to 15 miles, with 20-milers thrown in the several weeks before a marathon). ALL of those miles were run at my anaerobic threshhold, a pace under 6:00 per mile. I maintained a style of tempo running on a daily basis, achieving hard and easy efforts primarily by varying the distance I ran, although I could also vary the pace by as much as 30 seconds per mile. My training log shows that the first year my average pace per mile went above 6:00 was 1990. That average included wind-downs, before races, recovery days, after races, and recovery days after a multitude of running related injuries (my failure to stretch through much of this period led to many hamstring injuries).

I still run "tempo" pace, though it is now in the high 7's, and the distance I am able to cover is more likely 3 to 5 miles instead of 7 to 10. I continue to enjoy running and feel so much better after I achieve the discipline of a training run than I do on the days I am unable to fit running into my schedule.

FA50: Thank you Norm, you are truly an inspiration to all of us!

If Norm can accomplish so much after 50, then maybe we can benefit from a little exercise and an improved lifestyle, too, by finding a sport (or fitness activity) that we can train for and enjoy.

The Other Runner From Austin

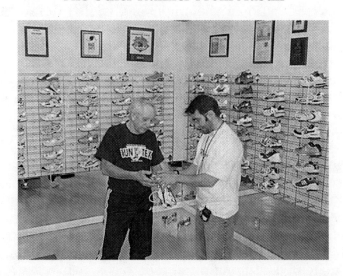

When **James Hill** of Austin, Texas took up running, at age 54, he was an overweight couch potato on high blood pressure medicine. Seven years later he holds the 60-64-age-group marathon record for the United States Corporate Athletics Association with a time of 3:08:30 (beating the old record by almost 10 minutes). His personal bests in the 5K, 18:26, and the 10K, 38:54 are equally impressive and competitive with many 30-something medal contenders.

We can learn a great deal from James about how to go from unfit to fit. Let's just listen to what he has to say (oh, the other runner from Austin, with a sub-4-hour marathon in his late forties, now resides at 1600 Pennsylvania Avenue).

FA50: James, what was your fitness level when you began running seven or so years ago?

James: When I started running about seven years ago, I was about thirty pounds overweight. I was also taking blood pressure medicine. My typical after-work activities were to go to the nearest Seven Eleven and get a Tall Boy, go home and drink three or four more, eat, and go to bed. I did not play golf or do anything except mow the grass every so often. I could only jog a quarter of a mile without stopping.

FA50: To what do you attribute your excellent running times: Exercise, diet, supplements, a specific training regimen, a mindset, a combination of these things, ...?

James: Let me first say that I was a slow runner in my younger days. The approach that I took was by accident, I believe, in the beginning. I decided that I needed to do something with my life. I decided to try running to see if I liked it. My first run was late one night because I did not want any of my neighbors to see me trying to run. I was able to run one quarter of a mile at a very slow rate. I had to stop and walk. When I recovered I then would run again as far as I could. The first goal I set was to be able to run one mile without stopping. In about a week I was able to do it. I then set a goal of three miles. This took a little longer, but it came.

What really got me running competitively was when I entered a 5K local race and finished third in my age group. I decided right then and there that I was going to win the next race I entered and I did. I really did not know any of the other runners to ask for help, so I bought four or five books on running. They all stated that you need an aerobic base and speed work. After a few months I met Paul Carrozza, the owner of Run-Tex, a running shoe store in Austin. I told him that I really enjoyed running and did not like for anyone in my age group to beat me. He invited me to train with one of his training groups. He recommended that I train with the advanced training group. The reason was that the younger runners would tend to pull me along and thus I would improve. His advice soon paid off and my times in the local races improved. I often would place in the top group. I still train with this group.

I do not take any drug-enhancing supplements. About the only change in my diet is that I do not drink beer anymore. My weight doesn't vary more than a couple of pounds from week to week. Within six months after taking up running my doctor took me off the blood pressure medicine.

FA50: Do you think that the average 50-plus-year-old can get in better shape than the average 20-or-30-year-old? Can everyday Joes (and Jameses) get fitter after 50 than they were before?

James: I definitely believe that I am in better shape than the average 20 to 30-year-old. This is based upon my ability to outrun a lot of younger runners. I believe that if the average 50-plus-year-old is in good health, he/she can get into better shape than the average 20 to 30-year -old person. I do believe, though, that a fit 30-year-old will outrun the equally-"fit" 50-year-old. I am not sure when I will start losing speed. If I continue to train the way I am training now, I do not see why I cannot run at my present level for another ten years or so. This is, unless I get injured.

FA50: What fringe benefits have you received from your Masters running?

James: Some of the fringe benefits I have definitely received from my running the last seven years are:

- I lowered my blood pressure and no longer take medicine.
- I lost 30 pounds of weight. I am 5'11", 165 pounds, 61 years old.
- I have met numerous new friends.
- I have traveled more in the last 5 years than I traveled in the previous thirty. My wife and I have made trips to runs in a lot of places — San Diego, Washington, DC, New York, Boston 5 times, Orlando, Santa Barbara, Los Gatos, Tucson, and LasVegas.
- I definitely stay charged and seem to have much more energy than most people my age.

As far as other health benefits, I do not have to take any type of medication.

FA50: Do you have any interesting stories related to your running that you would like to share?

James: A few years ago I was asked to run on a company, Southwestern Bell Telephone, relay team. This was a three person half marathon relay. About a week before the race, the person who had asked me to run came to me and said that they had picked another runner in my place. I asked him why and he told me that the other two team members, who were in their early 30s, thought I was too old. I thanked him for telling me the truth and assured him that I would outrun all three of the SOB's. I did, by 15 minutes.

FA50: What is a typical workout schedule like for you?
James:
Monday - I work out with a group of runners in Austin under the direction of a coach. We usually run a warm-up of two miles. We do different warm-up drills and then some kind of tempo (changing speeds) run or hill repeats. This is usually three to six miles. Then we run a two-mile cool down.

Tuesday - Three to six miles in my subdivision at about an eight-minute easy pace.

Wednesday - With the group in Austin, we run a warm up of between two and five miles, drills on the track. Our normal track workout is different speeds for a total of from 5,000 to 10,000 meters. Two-mile cool down.

Thursday - Three to eight miles in my subdivision at about an eight minute, easy pace.

Friday - Same as Thursday.

Saturday - Three to twenty-three miles in my subdivision or the longer runs on rural roads at about an eight minute easy pace. Based on what my training goal is, I often run up to 23 miles. This is not often, but about a month before I run a marathon, I get in long runs between 18 and 23 miles.

Sunday - Three to six miles in my subdivision at about an eight-minute, easy pace. I try to run every day, but there are very few weeks when I am able to do this. My plan is to miss a day each week — even though it is scheduled. My three to six-mile runs vary week to week. I often will increase my total distance for a few weeks and then lower the distance. My average weekly distance is between 50 and 60 miles; that's approximately seven or eight hours of running on a normal week.

FA50: What is your diet like? Is it extreme or Spartan-like to get so much out of a 61-year-old body?
James:
Breakfast - For the last 10 years or so I have been having 3 bananas and orange juice mixed in a blender — around 44 ounces

Lunch - This really varies. My wife and I eat out a lot. A normal meal may be: a serving of fish (three small catfish filets); a serving of pinto beans; french fried potatoes; and cole slaw. We eat a similar meal about once a week with barbecue instead of fish. About once a week I will eat at a cafeteria and usually have three servings of vegetables, salad, and bread (no meat). I do not eat dessert at noon.

Evening Meal - This is usually a smaller meal which will often be only a serving of mixed fruit. We also eat soup for the evening meal once a week or so. I often have dessert after the evening meal; a serving of ice cream or Jello would probably be the norm. Also, I often eat an orange, banana, or apple before going to bed (or some time during the day). I very seldom eat what I consider Fast Food. I have been taking a multi-vitamin for about the last year. I thought it might help me in case I am not getting everything I need in my meals.

FA50: What would you like to tell 50, 55, or 60-year-olds thinking about starting a running or fitness program? What is the best advice you could give them?

James: The best advice that I will and have often given others is that you have to set yourself a short-term goal. By setting a short-term goal, something that you can honestly measure, you will gain confidence and this will lead to more challenging goals that will make you stretch more and achieve more. This is where the individual will really start to see positive results. It is my belief that if one sets realistic goals that are reachable, the majority of the time he will meet or beat them.

Having a workout partner is also very helpful. Both of you will gain from the experience and it will surprise you how many new friends you will have before you know it. Some of my best and most loyal friends are ones I have met while running during the last four or so years.

FA 50: High blood pressure medicine and other medications can be expensive, as well as often having unpleasant side effects. By taking up a fitness-producing activity, like James did, we can eliminate or reduce our reliance on drugs, put some excitement back in our life, and fatten our wallet, all at the same time.

Staying Fit Under Duress

Denver and Nora Fox, in their sixties, are dealing with stressors most of us will fortunately never have to tackle. They could easily use their unique family situation as an excuse not to take care of themselves (i.e., eat right and exercise); instead they use their challenge as a reason why they need to be fitter than the average American. Here's their story, as told by Denver, in answer to our questions:

As the parents of two profoundly handicapped children, my wife and I have developed a number of techniques to help counter the intense stresses associated with the social, educational, medical, and other systems that are supposedly designed to assist us with our situation, but which, in fact, are often the source of intense problems, not solutions. First among these stress control techniques has been regular exercise. Over the years, we have consistently, on a daily basis, engaged in exercise of some sort. Even during intensive multi-month hospital stays, while supporting our sons on an 18-hour-per-day or more hospital and rehabilitation regimen, we have learned that if we don't exercise in some way or another, our health degenerates markedly.

As for food intake, that is our major nemesis. We both love to eat and weight is a constant battle. Also, for both of us, stress heightens our need to eat. As we have lived an extremely stressful life at times, sometimes the eating has gone out of control. If we charted our weight gains and losses, they would correlate directly with stress levels! We are totally aware of nutrition and appropriate eating techniques, and when in a stable stress environment, do pretty well. We eat little, if any, red meats and tend to keep saturated, trans-fatty acids and partially hydrogenated fats to a low level. We do lots of veggies and I love fruits. Protein comes in skinless chicken, nuts, and an occasional egg. We drink only skim milk. BUT, I love ice cream - it is truly my nemesis. Neither of us drinks any alcohol. I use no caffeine, and my wife may have a small sip of caffeine a couple of times per week. Neither of us has ever smoked.

I am approaching 61-years-old and my wife is 63. Over the years, our major exercise has been the simplest — walking. We generally walk briskly three to four miles daily on beautiful trails near our home. In addition, I took up biking three years ago and my wife two years ago. I used to do some running, but found that my knees were hurting and I stopped.

I have recently started a new full-time job, and it has significantly reduced my exercise, particularly during the first 10 weeks of the job. I now feel that I am in a position to get back into more exercise, as I have learned the intricacies of the job and can settle into a better routine.

As to accomplishments: I can ride 100 miles a day on my bike and have ridden two "Ride the Rockies" — bike trips through the Rockies of about seven days over many Colorado mountain passes and several centuries [100 mile rides]. Nora joined me for a portion of the Ride the Rockies this last year. I ocassionally (in the warm months) ride my bike to work (either 18 or 28 miles one way) and will do so regularly come Spring. I do some swimming and would like to do more.

I do resistive exercises, working out two to three times weekly. I have bench pressed 225 pounds. I work out at home, about an hour per session. I can do 10 chin-ups in a row. I know that when I exercise, my endorphins really do come into play — I feel great after a workout. I am definitely fitter now than when I was 30!

Denver and Nora take care of themselves because of the stress in their lives; not in spite of it. They owe it to their two profoundly-handicapped children, who depend on them, to stay healthy and fit. In light of the Foxes' family life situation, are our excuses valid or just convenient. Maybe we can get in shape *for* our loved ones who count on us.

A Sterling Example of Fitter After 50

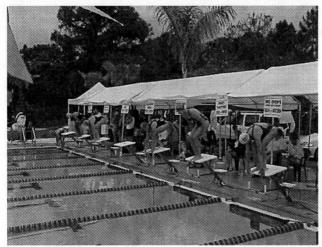

Jean Sterling, third swimmer from the right, at nationals

Jean Sterling shows us how to be fitter after 50. Here is her interview:

FA50: To what do you attribute your superior well-being (e.g., diet, exercise, relaxation techniques, spiritual pursuits, ...)?

Jean: I think the exercise comes first. Eating right follows right along with the exercise program because if I don't eat right, I feel blah the next day and don't feel like exercising.

FA50: What "proof" of your fitness do you have (e.g., endurance race scores, percentage of body fat, anecdotal stories)?

Jean: I ran my first marathon when I was 49 and did my best time for the marathon when I was 51 (4:48). In my fifties I did triathlons, including some of the Olympic distance (1.5K swim, 40K bike, and 10K run). For the past five years or so I have concentrated mostly on swimming and have made the National top-10 list in the breaststroke, butterfly, freestyle, and individual medley. I am most proud of my personal records. My most recent personal record was in the 50 butterfly just two weeks ago (I am now 63 years old). In my late 50s I set personal records for the 200 individual medley and the 400 individual medley, swimming better times than I had done in my 40s. This year I swam the 200-meter butterfly for the first time and my stroke held up to the end of the race [the fly takes more energy and strength than the other strokes and 200 meters is a long distance to do the butterfly]. The time I did may or may not make this year's top-ten list — the competition gets better and better every year. [Note: Since Jean's interview, she was ranked #1 on the 2001 national top ten list for the long course 200 individual medley for her new age group (65-69) — way to go Jean!]

Before I started exercising in my forties, I had put on weight like most people do — I weighed 162 (and it wasn't muscle, either). I am now down to 139 (and a lot of what I lost was fat). At the doctor's last week, my resting heart rate was 49! I am MUCH fitter than I was 20 years ago and most likely fitter than the average 20-year-old.

FA50: What challenges have you overcome?

Jean: Taking off the blubber I had accumulated. It took a lot of gumption for me to go out and try to run when I weighed 162 — I really felt like a spectacle.

FA50: Can you give a sample of your regular workouts and/or diet?

Jean: I will share two interval swim workouts that I have done recently.

1. 500 easy
16 x 25 on 30 seconds — Alternate freestyle and another stroke
   pull 500
   2 x (100 fly + 200 back +100 free) on 9 minutes
   8 x 50 backstroke on 1:10
   10 x 50 freestyle on 1 minute
   200 easy

2. 500 easy
20 x 25 individual medley order (fly, back, breast, free) on 40 sec.
   pull 4 x 200 freestyle on 4 minutes
   2 x (100 butterfly + 200 breaststroke + 100 freestyle) on 9 minutes

8 x 50 backstroke on 1:10
10 x 50 freestyle on 1 minute
200 easy.

FA50: Makes me tired just thinking about workouts like these. They'd have to keep filling the pool because of all the water I would swallow. Anyway, what would you like people to know about you? What can people learn from you — your experiences?

Jean: They can learn that if they get started and don't get sidetracked, that they can become fit and more healthy. I don't know if exercise makes you live longer, but for sure it makes you live better. It's a real joy to feel good.

FA 50: Thank you, Jean. You are an inspiration to all of us.

If Jean can swim those impressive, exhausting-sounding interval workouts, then surely we can put in a few laps at the local pool on a regular basis (if we can swim, that is). If not, there is always the old stand-by — long walks.

Once An Athlete, Always An Athlete

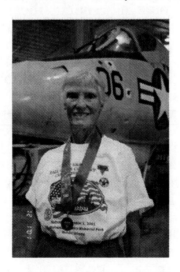

Ruth Anderson has been an athlete just about all her life. As a young lady in high school she enjoyed basketball, field hockey, volleyball, and tennis; her college years were filled with basketball and tennis. Unlike most of us, she continued her active lifestyle as an adult, first with tennis and swimming and then gradually switching over to just running. Now in her early 70s, the former scientist at the Lawrence Livermore Labs in California shows us that we don't have to give up athletic competition just because our life's work demands a large chunk of our time and energy.

Through the years, Ruth has shown a versatility rare in runners. Runners tend to stick with a small range of distances to concentrate on, specializing in anything from being strictly sprinters to milers and 1500-meter specialists to 5-and-10K racers to marathoners and finally to ultra-marathoners. In sharp contrast to this inclination toward specialization, Ruth has competed in *and set records in* everything from 800 meter "sprints" to 24-hour, ultra-marathon endurance race/events.

Here is just a little sampling of what Ruth has accomplished in her long and illustrious running career. At age 50, she set a US record at the 1979 50-mile championships in Houston, Texas with a time of 7 hours, 10 minutes and "change." My calculations indicate that that averages out to 8:37 per mile *for 50 miles.* Having struggled to complete just a 10K race (6 miles at an 8-minute-per-mile pace), at age 54, on a hot and humid day, on a hilly course (those are my excuses for not going faster), I have a *sense* of what Ruth had to overcome and of the remarkable nature of her accomplishment. In 1986, at 57, she set a 24-hour track record of 110.5 miles. She won the 5K Championships, in Carlsbad, California, in 1995, then 65, with an impressive time of 26:14.

Ruth's love of running has not only kept her on the track all these years, but also behind the scenes, too. She has worked on committees and in administrative positions to advance the roles and opportunities of women in running and Masters running. She was instrumental in getting the women's marathon event into the Olympic Games and women competitors in the London-to-Brighton 54.2-mile-ultra-marathon, among other accomplishments. For these and other efforts, she received national awards from the USATF for meritorious service in 1977, 1984, and 1991. Among her other awards and honors are the Runner's World Nurmi Award for being the Best USA Woman Ultra-marathoner in 1978, at the age of 49; the best Masters runner; and induction into the Road Runner's Club of America Hall of Fame (one of the first two women to receive this honor). At this writing, she was still competing as well as organizing teams of older runners to compete in relays.

During our communications, Ruth happened to mention that she hasn't "had a cold for years." Another time she said, "I know how lucky I am about the lack of colds, flu, etc, over the years!" Now remember, she's doing a lot of traveling to compete and serve on committees, etc.; oh, and I forgot to mention, she's also run in more than 100 marathons and more than 70 ultra-marathons (i.e., 24-hour races, 50-milers, etc.). The question is, how has she stayed so well in light of the fact that stress depresses the immune system, opening the way for bacteria and viruses to take hold? Twenty-four-hour races, as well as competing in any long distance race (never mind the elite level) has to be a major stress on the body. Why has Ruth fared so well while those of us all around her are coming down with colds, flu, etc. Ruth confesses that, "[I] Don't really know why so much good *luck*. Sorry, not much of an answer." That said, here's what she did come up with:

1. By upping her Vitamin C, she has escaped colds.
2. Not being around children lessens her exposure to cold germs.
3. She's never been an overtrainer. Through the years, "I only did 55-60 mile [weekly] averages." In 1974 she tried 70 miles in preparation for the International Women's Marathon in Germany, but found it made her too tired to perform well. Ruth doesn't believe in mega-training. Now in her seventies, Ruth says she's "lucky to do 40 miles."
4. Ruth uses good recovery practices, but doesn't seem to need as much rest as some competitors after major competitions.
5. She's not compulsive about her running (i.e., doesn't train when not feeling up to it).
6. She eats well, a good variety of health-supporting foods. To quote Ruth, "Pastas

are high on the list of common food, but do try to balance it with proteins, including red meat along with lots of fish and foul. I am particularly fond of yogurt, fruit of all kinds, and more selective on vegetables. Do drink beer and wine, mostly with meals, and love dark chocolate, to name a 'weakness' or two."

7. Was taking Vitamin E before it became fashionable, vitamin C, desiccated liver (for iron), and a multi-vitamin. Did this as health insurance due to all the travel and extra-long running (competitions) although "really do think I get enough of most of these in my diet."

Although any or all these practices may have kept the cold viruses, flu bugs, etc. at bay, my theory is that it is Ruth's love and enthusiasm for the sport of running that has kept her well above all else. For when we are excited, enthusiastic, joyful, and love what we are doing, stress is minimized and the immune system is fortified. We'll talk more about this in future chapters.

Ruth has attained this astonishing level of radiant health and great athletic accomplishments with an average of just over an hour a day of running. We know for a fact that we also can have exceptional fitness and health (maybe not world-class caliber) with just 3 hours of aerobic and strength workouts each week. That's just 6 half-hour sessions a week for optimal well-being. By giving up just 3 hours of mind-numbing, Alzheimer's-disease-attracting TV (some research is pointing that way) per week, we can reap benefits similar to Ruth's. If Ruth can run 24-hour races, then we can at least _____ _____.

Challenge Your Limits

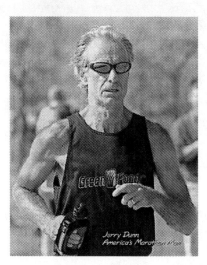

"Don't limit your challenges ... Challenge your limits!" **Jerry Dunn**, America's Marathon Man, has lived by these words. As a result, in the year 2000, Jerry, then 54 years old, ran and completed *200 marathons*, an unofficial world record. It's safe to say that Jerry is fitter after 50 because when he first started running, at age 30, in 1976, "a quarter-mile run on the beach was about as much as I could do ... or wanted to do ..., but mostly, COULD do." At the time Jerry says he was "at the peak of my drinking and drugging days."

Let's take a look at some significant aspects of Jerry's life, and at what has made him, in his fifties, "the most durable long distance runner on the planet." Here it is in Jerry's own words (with some editing):

Watching my 47-year-old father die of a heart attack had more impact on my young teenage mind than I was able to comprehend at the time it happened ... or even for many years to come. That one afternoon, in 1964, altered the course of my life dramatically ... and not all for the good.

He was young. He looks a lot younger through 54-year-old eyes than he did through ones that were only 18. He was fat — 255 pounds; at 5 foot 11 inches that's fat! He smoked two to three packs of Pall Malls a day. He wasn't lazy, but exercise to him was washing the car or mowing the lawn or sending me down to the drugstore on my bike to get a couple more packs of cigarettes. I guess you could say that he wasn't the type of father that you would expect to have sired America's Marathon Man — the most durable runner on the planet.

My journey through life from December 4, 1964 to December 10, 2000, the day I completed my personal "Mission Impossible" [200 marathons in one year], can be compared to the Biblical story of the Prodigal Son. I spent a lot of years running from and now I'm running to ... What I was running from is pretty obvious, but what I'm running toward is where the inspiration for others may lie.

The act of running moves us forward toward something — either the finish line of a race; the end of our allotted distance for that day's training run; or maybe toward home where we started. But running is about movement and when we can consistently move toward a goal, whatever it may be, we are putting ourselves into the "flow" of life and from my vantage point that's an exciting place to be.

As with most everything else in our lives, the transition from drinking to abstinence was a process. When I first began running, I was still drinking, smoking some cigarettes, and doing quite a bit of marijuana. There was also an occasional line of cocaine, as long as it was free (I would never purchase "coke" because then I would have REALLY been a drug user/abuser). The beer that I consumed during this "overlap" period was a great source of carbohydrates...RIGHT (every alcoholic has a ready rationale for his/her "condition"). Anyway, for the first 6 or 7 years that I ran, I continued to "use." I remember one morning in particular I arrived at the start line of a race very hung over, having slept about three hours, with the too-many-cigarettes-the-night-before taste in my mouth and wondering "what in the hell am I doing here?" The worst part of the whole experience was that I did fairly well in the race and was therefore able to continue fooling myself into thinking that I was "Superman" — able to do anything.

In the months prior to my first marathon, in 1981, I had reduced my drinking considerably. The reduction in consumption was due in part to my training, but I was also making very little money at the time and couldn't afford to drink much. I realize that a serious alcoholic does not let a lack of funding deter him from his drinking, but besides not having much money, I was also trying to patch up my second marriage.

My running and my marathon training had not yet taken on addictive proportions, but the time spent out on the roads was filling up time that I had formerly spent drinking. In those early days I was an evening runner, the time of day I used to spend in bars or drinking at home. So it occupied my time; therefore, I wasn't drinking as much. My running, also, began to transform my self-image. As I drank less and ran more, I was able to say, "Yeah, I'm trainin' for a marathon." I began to see myself less and less as an alcoholic and more and more as a runner; and I liked "runner" better ... I liked myself better.

Here are some more insightful tidbits about "America's Marathon Man" and what he has to teach us:

1. STRETCHING - *When I first began running and until I started running ultra-marathons, in 1989, I always stretched before training runs and races. During those years I was still working on improving my "race pace" and my speed in general. I was quite aware of the importance of "warming up" the muscles before a hard training run or race. But when I began to run longer distances, at a slower pace, in a less competitiive atmosphere, I found that the first couple of miles worked just fine as a way to warm up. In other words, a 20-mile training run at a 9:30 pace is a whole lot different than a 10-mile training run at a 7:00 minute pace.*

As far as any stretching during my 200 in 2000 — it didn't happen. Prior to starting the year I had considered establishing a quick warm-up routine, but never got it started. There were a few days during the year that I would arrive back at my car and put both hands on the roof and alternately stretch out each leg for a few seconds, but you could probably count the times I did that on the fingers of my two hands.

In summary, I don't stretch before or after running. I don't "walk it off" either; and I don't typically jump into a Jacuzzi or hot tub .... 99% of the time my routine is to finish a run, whether it be a training run or a marathon, and just move on to the next task at hand. That could be catching a plane to get home; sitting down at the computer; making breakfast for me and my wife; or whatever is next on the day's agenda. I guess running is SUCH a normal part of my daily routine that I don't feel a need to treat it much differently than doing the laundry, grocery shopping, or going to work.

Even though I don't stretch myself, I DO strongly recommend that beginning runners, and those runners who are still in the "competitive" phase of their running career, spend some time stretching both before and after a training run or a race.

2. EATING - Jerry tries to eat 5 or 6 small, but "nutritious" meals a day; a typical day might look like this:

5:15 - Barley Essence nutritional supplement — Powdered barley in water

5:30 - A cup of coffee

7:00 - Oatmeal, milk, banana, brown sugar, & orange juice

10:00 - PowerBar High Protein Bar & water

12:00 - Tuna/beef/chicken, salad, bread, & water ...sometimes apple pie

2:00 - Fruit smoothie with Endurox R4 (supplement)

5:30 - Pork/chicken/beef/fish, corn, green beans, bread & water

8:00 - Popcorn, salted; apple and cheese

Jerry says, "*I tend to say that I eat whatever I want, which is basically true. However, after many years of dietary experimentation, my wants are most often in a nutritionally healthy spectrum. I have my McDonald's attacks; my Haagen Daz days; and I can't eat a BLT without chips. So, I'm far from the purist status of many eaters, but as with everything else in life, there's a balance.*

3. SUPPLEMENTING - Since March of 1993, Barley Essence from Green Foods has been the first thing in his system each and every morning. Jerry says that the benefits are that it "... helps me maintain a high level of energy; fights inflammation (from overuse of muscles - go figure; and supplies me with the 'Green' I need in my diet." It is the only "dietary supplement" that he takes. The only other supplement he takes is a recovery drink, Endurox R4. He puts 2 scoops of this in his afternoon smoothie, as well as using it on long training runs of 10 miles or more. Its purpose is to reduce muscle soreness, replenish glycogen stores, re-hydrate the system, and restore depleted protein and carbohydrates.

4. VISUALIZATION - *On a daily basis, during last years' adventure [200 marathons in 2000], I used visualization to*

break up the 26.2 mile distance by looking ahead in my mind to one of the "landmarks" that I had established along the marathon route. For instance, in January, in Carlsbad, there was a tall smoke stack at mile 4.5 that wasn't perceptually visible until I made the turn at mile 2 and came out onto the coastline. But in my mind's eye I could see it when I left the starting line at the shopping mall parking lot and it drew me up that first hill past the sidewalk flower stand, that opened most mornings at 6:15, and then out on to the boulevard that bounds the ocean and then on to the smoke stack. The next landmark was the turnaround at 7 miles, at which point I was afforded a vista-type view of the ocean and the flower fields below.

Just as I needed to visualize myself finishing each day's run, I also found it extremely helpful to break each day's run into chunks. I also realized on about day 4 or 5, that even though I needed to think positvely about being able to do 200 of "these things," it was important to take the project one day at a time — one portion of each day at a time.

Other times I consciously visualized myself as "one with the universe"...really. You know, goin' with the flow. Running as though I were meant to be out in the streets of LA, in rush hour traffic on a Friday morning. The point is that I saw myself as vital to the overall scheme of things at that particular time and in that particular place.

As for visualization being part of the preparation for my daily marathon, I guess the most frequent image I used was that of me running, period. There were many days that I had to force myself to get started and on those days, if I told myself, "you can do this, you wanna do this, you're going to reach your goal if you get out there today and run"; and then pictured myself a few miles into it, I was on my way to another "daily victory."

5. INJURIES AND SICKNESS - Jerry has had no serious injuries or sickness in his almost 50,000 miles/25-years of running. He has had his share of minor ailments, such as turned ankles, pulled muscles, abrasions from falls, and a summer of shin splints. His only illnesses have been an occasional cold and one notable bout with the flu. For a cold he usually takes a couple of days off and rests; but if he's in the middle of one of his multi-day runs he'll down some cold medicine and keep chugging. Concerning his coming down

with the flu, he says, "The first week of 1993, as I was just beginning my quest for 93 in '93,' I got a horrendous case of the flu and had to run a couple of pretty 'unpleasant' marathons." Let's just say it's a rarity for Jerry to get ill.

6. GENETICS - *In my case, I think the major portion of my success is due to training, diet, and the mental approach. I have a tiny, non-athletic mother and I had an overweight, non-athletic dad, so I don't think I've got a helluva lot goin' on for me genetically. Unless, of course, you consider tenacity, bullheadedness, independence, and humility to be genetically transferable. And I agree with Helen Klein [see chapter 3] -- it's way more mental than it is physical. I mean, you can only get in so "gooda" shape and after that you have to "want it!"* Genetically speaking, Jerry is 6 foot 1 inch tall and weighs 152 (although at age 30 he weighed in at 165 pounds).

7. TIREDNESS - *I don't immediately recall any days that I actually felt energized at the end of 26.2 [miles]. There were days when I had a feeling of excitement, I guess you could say. Like day 77 when I hit 2,000 miles; day 100 when I was halfway to my goal; and, of course, day 200, having reached my goal. I really can't say I was often "fatigued" after a few consecutive days of marathon runs either. Tired? Yes.*

Another "mental" aspect of how I felt at the end of my "work day" was that I was often "thankful" to be finished with another one. And in that feeling of prayerful thankfulness I found a kind of physical resting space. Like that first night's sleep at home, in your own bed, after 2 or 3 weeks on the road. You know, like..."man am I glad to be here!"

8. REST AND RECUPERATION - During his 200 in 2000, Jerry would run a marathon each day for about the first 17 days of the month and then he would rest and recuperate for a couple of weeks before starting the cycle all over again. Not only that, but each run lasted "just" 4 or 5 hours leaving him 19 or 20 hours to rest up. After he finished his 200th marathon on December 10, 2000 he took the rest of the month off from ANY running, starting up again on January 1. Jerry knows that sufficient rest is a critical part of any endurance activity.

9. JERRY'S ADVICE TO BOOMERS - *Be honest with yourself about WHY you want to get back in shape. ... it's popular among us 50-somethings, us Boomers, to get on the fitness bandwagon,*

and if that's why you're "getting in shape" — it aint gonna work. But, when YOU have made the decision and the committment that YOU want to feel better, look better, live better/longer and more energetically, then and only then will the transformation be successful.

Part of me balks at the idea of "advising" people on how to get fit. My tendency is to believe that if they want to, they will. And part of the process of committing to "getting fit" is the personal investigation and experimentation into how to make that happen. I think I'm more of an "encourager" than I am an "instructor" or fitness guru. There are plenty of those already out there with their books and their tapes and their diet plans and their charts for measuring this and that; and I'd say most of them are based on solid and successful concepts. So I don't really have any new, secret formula for getting fit. What I do have to offer is the slogan that a lot of us "old drunks" live by, and that is — keep it simple. Being fit, being well, being happy is not all that complicated; getting there can be a bitch/real struggle — but once we're there, "fit is fun."

I think the average 50-year-old, or person of any age for that matter, can look at my "progressive" successes and draw inspiration from them in the following way. They can, first of all, realize that it's been a process from that first quarter mile on the beach to 5,240 miles in one year, the time span is 25 years. So that 50-year-old has to understand that you don't just "git fit" overnight. Second, even though the "steps" in my progression of [running] successes have sometimes been giant steps, like running across one state in 1990, to running across 12 states in in'91, [to 104 marathons in 1993, at age 47, in honor of his father who died at 47], *they have been carefully calculated to be within my personal range of feasability.* Put more succinctly, know yourself, push yourself, but do it within the bounds of your own capabilities. Too many people limit themselves with hindering beliefs, such as "I'm too old for that." *DON'T LIMIT YOUR CHALLENGES — CHALLENGE YOUR LIMITS!*

In our next chapter we'll meet some individuals, most of them in their seventies, eighties, and yes, nineties, who have extended the prime of life well beyond the usual 50 or so years.

CHAPTER 3 IF THEY CAN DO IT, ... THE PRIME-OF-LIFERS -

70s, 80s & 90s

What can we learn from a 75-year-old grandmother who runs 100-mile races; a fitness instructor and amateur contortionist in her late eighties; a 91-year-old swimmer who swims 1 mile in trainings; and an eighty-something world-class sprinter? We can learn that vibrant well-being abounds at all ages and that we CAN not only be fitter after 50, but also, after 70, 80 and 90. Now let's meet these amazing enjoyers of life and find out why they have so much more vitality and vigor and why they are so much more "alive" than the great majority of their peers.

If Grandma Can Do It ...

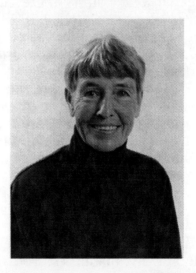

At 53, in 1976, she was an emergency room nurse and mother of four, who had *never* entered nor had any interest in the athletic arena. Two years later, retired from the ER, she was cajoled by her husband, Norman, into accompanying him in a 10-mile race; a competition which she didn't enjoy at all until she crossed the finish line — in last place at that.

But wait! In 1982, at the age of 59, she entered the Hawaiian Ironman Triathlon (the epic swim, bike, and run-a-marathon competition). In 1989, now a 66-year-old grandmother of 9, she completed the Grand Slam of 100-mile mountain-trail runs (the Vermont 100, the Wasatch 100, Colorado's Leadville 100, and the Western States 100); plus one more to grow on, the Angeles Crest 100, all in just a 16-week time period. In 1995, in her prime at 72, she ran the Marathon Des Sables, a grueling 145-mile stage race across the Sahara Desert in Morocco; then just 2 weeks later (with hardly time to catch her breath), she competed in AND finished the first annual Eco Challenge, in Utah, a 370-mile multi-sport, multi-day, race (including horseback riding, canoeing, and rock climbing — 1200-foot vertical cliffs) in which over half the competitors (most just half her age) could not complete this rugged event.

Who is this marvel? Her name is **Helen Klein**. Helen makes us reexamine our old, outdated beliefs about aging. Helen proudly says to us, through her actions and awe-inspiring accomplishments, that the decline we associate with getting older may be highly exaggerated — to our detriment.

Helen has unquestionably become fitter after 50. She can show us what gave her 23 injury and illness-free years of competition, years in which she set more than 75 age-group, American and world records. These included her 100-mile world record — 21:03:01 (21 hours and 3 minutes); her 54 marathons and 130 ultra-marathons (including 5 and 6-day race events); her winning the coveted Arete Award for courage in sports; and her being named *Runner's World magazine's* Woman of the Century (100-mile racing, that is).

Let's look at how an un-athletic Helen Klein went from emergency-room nurse to world-champion athlete, all after the age of 55. Like many readers of this book, maybe even you, before that first 10-mile race, Helen didn't like the idea of getting all sweaty from running. She was so embarrassed by just the idea of her neighbors and friends (yes, and even total strangers) seeing her running around town, that she had her husband measure out a one-fifth mile "track" in their backyard where she could run in relative obscurity, in preparation for that first 10-miler. In addition, she thought that running a race was a crazy way for one to spend his or her time; and she regarded walking as a plenty good means of locomotion. However, once she commits to something, anything, even something as insane as giving Norm her word that she would train for and run a 10-mile race with him, there is no turning back.

Her first training session, she could only do two laps around the homemade track, and she told me, "I thought I would die!" The next day she added another lap and found that it was not quite so exhausting. With this experience, she decided to add a lap each day for the several weeks of training. In 10 weeks Helen was ready for the race. She and her husband, Norm, completed the 10-mile race in 2 hours (a 12-minute-mile pace), not exactly a gold medal performance. But, she did get a T-shirt, a trophy (she was the only woman in her age-group), and her picture in the paper (crossing the finish line), which she thought was "cool." Most importantly, she experienced the satisfaction of having completed a difficult challenge.

Norm wanted to keep racing and so Helen sort of got dragged into the running scene, first as a cheerleader for her husband and then as a runner herself (if you are going to be at the races, you might as well run in them — it makes the time go faster). Eventually she got caught up in the challenge of seeing if she could run this distance and that distance; this race and that race, with their differing obstacles and challenges; and "viola`!" a world champion was born. But, why the great success?

1. Before she ran in a race, she had to have the belief that she could possibly do it. Helen says it this way, "Before I tackle something, I have to believe in my heart and mind that there is a possibility of finishing; then I give it my best."

2. Helen focused on the camaraderie of the race, the excitement and the sense of accomplishment she would have when she crossed the finish line. This focus develops a strong desire. In Helen's words, "When you really, really want something, you have just taken the first step in making it happen. You have given yourself permission to succeed."

3. Next, once she had the belief and desire, she took the action steps necessary to make it happen. She registered for the event, got the airline tickets, and trained as needed.

4. Having trained properly and sufficiently, she then had the confidence critical to completing her goal — the race. Concerning this confidence, Helen has said, "When confidence is lost, doubt moves in. When doubt moves in your goal is given low priority in your mind. Move past doubt, and do what it takes to re-establish that confidence because it is there that you will find success."

5. Helen has been blessed with good genes and excellent biomechanics, but not great athletic or running ability. She tends to agree with the sports doctors who would say that the genes contribute only about 20% to performance.

6. Helen benefits from an excellent diet. She goes far beyond the recommended 5-a-day fruits and vegetables. Helen eats 5 or 6 fruits *and* 5 or 6 vegetables each day. She also enjoys whole grains, small four-ounce helpings of meat and/or fish and plenty of liquids. She stays away from junk foods and sodas. The only time she indulges in sodas/colas is during long races, using the carbs and caffeine as a pick-me-up. Interestingly, she reached her Hall-of-Fame status without any nutritional or herbal supplementation, not even a multi-vitamin. However, at 75, at the advice of Mr. Aerobics himself, Dr. Kenneth Cooper, she began taking anti-oxidants for the first time.

7. She started competing because she and Norm like to do things together. She continued because of the challenge; the awesome feeling of accomplishing feats of endurance that others considered impossible; and to experience that which stretches her to the limit.

8. While running, she focuses on keeping her body relaxed and her form good. The resulting

suppleness of her muscles keeps her injury and (to a point) stress free.

9. She stays positive as much as possible, focusing on her goal (the finish line) instead of the obstacles (snow, freezing rain, steep hills, ...). To help keep negative thoughts at bay, she uses mantras, such as "relax and move." Helen would have you understand that it really is "more mental than physical."

10. One of her weapons is the gratitude she feels. Helen says it this way, "Gratitude is such a beautiful word. When we have gratitude in our hearts for that which we do have instead of bitterness for what we don't have, the world becomes a place of smiles instead of frowns."

11. Helen's generosity, willingness, and desire to help others is yet another of her secrets to success. Her belief is that "the greatest gift we can give another is the gift of encouragement. Not only do I hope to encourage with my words, but also, by my example." The significance of this trait will be made clear in chapter 4.

Note: Don't mistakenly confuse these 100-mile races with 100 consecutive one-mile strolls in the park. Most of these are mountain-trail races (with the operative word being "mountain"). Rick Kerby of the Shenandoah Valley Runners' club in Virginia has experienced parts of the Leadville Trail 100, for example, and has this to say about it: *"This ultramarathon bills itself as 'The Race Across the Sky' as no part of the course is below 9,200 ft. elevation and runners summit 12,600 ft. Hope Pass twice during the run in a difficult (to put it mildly) 20-mile stretch ...with an air molecule density of 2 parts oxygen per every 4 square miles -- or so it felt... After mile 45, runners must climb Hope Pass for the first time — an ascent of 3,400 ft. in 3.5 miles — before descending 2,700 ft. in a tooth-rattling 2 miles to reach a turnaround in an abandoned mining town called Winfield. Then, they have to turn around and climb the same staggering 2,700 ft. in 2 miles to cross back over the pass on their way back. The Race Director is an evil, twisted sadist."* Now think about running five of these mountain-trail 100-milers in a 16-week period, like Helen did at age 66. Amazing, isn't it?

If great-grandma Helen can cover 373 miles during a 6-day race and climb 1200-foot sheer cliffs during a 370-mile eco-challenge, then maybe we can get up and moving, too. Why get moving? Helen would tell us, "Don't limit goals because of age or sex stereotypes ... [because] as soon as you begin to become inactive, you start to lose it." We can thank Helen for expanding the boundaries of what is possible for all of us. Now is our chance to learn from Helen and push the boundaries even wider.

Not Quite Ready For The Old Folks' Home

Don McNelly did not start running until age 48. Thirty-two years later, at age 79, he had run 560 marathons and ultra-marathons; that is nearing 600 races of 26 miles *or more* each. He's raced in all 50 states, each Canadian province and territory, and 20 countries. Most impressive to me is the fact that he has run 289 of his marathons/ultras since turning 70 (by my calculations that's an average of 32 races — *long* races — per year). And Don is not done yet. His next big goal is to complete his 600th in 2002. He's done all this despite having "always been too heavy and an unnatural athlete." Just imagine what he could have accomplished if he had possessed a Michael Jordan-type body. Probably not half as much; maybe none of it at all. As with all of us, his accomplishments grew out of his life experiences and his physical and mental attributes, both "good" and "bad."

Don ran his first marathon in Boston in 1969. After he got organized, he set out to break 4 hours for the marathon, which he did a few times. Then, as he matured as a runner, he switched from focusing on times to aiming to complete 100 marathons/ultras; then 200, 300, and eventually to today's 600 quest.

"...Our avocation is much more mental than physical," he wrote in *Marathon and Beyond* magazine. His advice, after 32 years of running experience, is to "...not be too hung up on how you are doing overall. In the long run, your health and ability to keep running is more important than the next PR [personal record]." Don has had to modify his goals as his circumstances have changed, as we all should learn to do. He's not nearly as fast as he once was, but then how many young adults can run 50 miles or even a single mile?

If Don can run 560 marathons/ultras, then we can set a goal to walk or run 100 total miles or ... in the next 6 or 12 months or we can ....

Seeing the Country In Retirement

It is not unusual for a retired couple to want to crisscross our great nation taking in small towns and big cities alike in an RV or motor-home. Seventy-three-year-old **Paul Reese** and his wife Elaine chose to add a little twist to this common scenario; in 1990 they decided to travel coast to coast, California to South Carolina, via their motor-home with *Paul running along behind* the vehicle. That's right, he resolved to traverse the 3,200 miles on foot, while his wife took care of the support and supply side of the proposition.

Paul ran a little over 26 miles per day (a marathon a day) for 122 straight days; plus 5 more ceremonial-miles on the first and last days for media coverage. Elaine would pull off the road every 3 miles and wait for Paul to catch up so she could feed him some of his daily requirement of 6,000 calories, keep him hydrated, and visit with/check on him. His secret weapons for accomplishing this exhausting, world-record-shattering marathon-of-marathons were this nourishment (the constant feedings) and the recovery phase (turning in each night shortly after supper). This allowed his 73-year-young body to have the energy and stamina to be on the road at 5:00 each morning, and to finally make it to their destination, Hilton Head, South Carolina, where as a highlight of the trip he *ran and jumped* into the Atlantic to celebrate the completion of this epic trek.

But, while this trip was very satisfying, it just wasn't enough. He wasn't satisfied to just cross the US; he wanted to cross each individual state — all 50. Hence, in subsequent summers, from the ages of 75 to 79, Paul proceeded to run across all the states west of the Mississippi; albeit, in a more leisurely fashion — only 21 miles each day and a slothful 7 AM start. He capped it all off by traversing the rest of the states, the ones east of the Mississippi, at the age of 80. In all Paul Reese traipsed 7,648 miles.

Why would anyone do this and more importantly, was it worth it? People like Paul take on this sort of adventure for the challenge and enjoyment of doing something unique and difficult, for the sense of accomplishment, for the stories garnered to tell others, and for a host of other reasons. This challenge with its adversities and hardships, among other things, helped the Reeses:

1. Reaffirm their belief in the existence of God
2. Renew their appreciation for the beauty of this country
3. Learn the lesson (and pass it along to others) of the importance of breaking major goals into smaller bite-size pieces

Paul has proved that older folks can accomplish far more than we formerly thought possible. Speaking about Paul's (and Elaine's) accomplishment Arnold Schwarzenegger said it was "a giant step forward regarding our concepts of aging." It will, he added, "awaken people in their 60s and 70s to their inherent capabilities."

Paul has writtten "... two keys to accomplishing a goal: believe you can do it, then be fully resolved to accomplish it and be unflinching in your resolve."

You may be thinking, "But he was obviously blessed with good health. My body has maladies, aches and pains, that prevent me from being able to exercise." Then maybe you should know that Paul suffered from and overcame prostate cancer, asthma, and a bad back (spondylolysis). Maybe you think, "that's fine, but I have arthritis or ... How can I possibly get the exercise I know I need?" Where there is a will there is a way. For example, some senior fitness champs with arthritis swim, as it is easier on their joints. Remember, one of the major recommendations of the "experts" is for those with arthritis, diabetes, osteoporosis, ... to exercise (of course, always check with your physician first if you have a malady such as these).

We don't have to walk from here to Kalamazoo or anywhere else; but if we want the thrill of taking our 6-year-old grandson to Disney World for the first time or our great-granddaughter to Six Flags, we need the energy and vigor to be able to walk the several miles it will take to cover these wonderlands for children (and remember, piggy-back rides may be an essential ingredient for optimal enjoyment, and I don't think *you* will be the one receiving the piggy-back ride!).

If Paul can run 122 consecutive daily marathons, then surely we can take a 30-minute walk/jog 3 times a week and/or do strength training at the local gym or in our basement 2 or 3 times week so that we can be part of and share our grandkids' and great-grandkids' joyous life experiences.

Portions of this story and the Don McNelly story were originally published in the September/October 2000 Issue of Marathon and Beyond. Reprinted with permission of 42K (+) Press, Inc. www.marathonandbeyond.com

A 21-Year Dance-A-Thon

Lenore Schaeffer fell in love with dancing when, at age 12, she fell in love with a dancer whom she later married. When he died an untimely death, she later married a man who couldn't dance for health reasons, so at 42 she put away her dancing shoes. At age 82, despite failing eyesight, she dusted off her dancing shoes and took up ballroom dancing — again.

Lenore won her first dancing awards in her eighties. Now, you might think that these were just the awards that are given to the youngest competitor because she is so cute and the oldest dancer (because she's still upright and can wobble across the floor for a few agonizing minutes), but they are not! These are prestigious ribbons and trophies where she beats out much younger competitors, such as the first place award Lenore won for fox trot and waltz in the Victor Dru International Invitational Contest in Las Vegas. In all she has won over 200 dancing awards, including a trophy at age 101.

Maybe you are thinking that the waltz is nice and slow and that's not such a big deal. You should know that she loves and performs the rumba, mambo, cha-cha, and even rock 'n' roll for audiences all across the fruited plain, including on the Tonight Show with Jay Leno. In order to keep up her strength and stamina, Lenore works out at her local gym on a regular basis, although in recent years she's cut back to once or twice a week.

If Lenore can dance competitively and perform past age 100, then WE CAN look into what dancing (or other activity) is available locally. There are ballroom dances (and lessons), square dances, tap, contra dances, line dances, aerobic dance, belly, and others in just about every town or city with a population sufficient to support them. Check them out. You are never too old a dog to learn new tricks and to enjoy the thrill of dancing. And who knows, you just might meet your soul mate — if you're not already hitched, that is. Or maybe you would just enjoy putting on some of your favorite music and dancing around in the privacy of your home.

Kids Just Ride Bikes, But Adults Cycle

What odds would you give a 55-year-old, overweight (245 pounds on an average-size frame), out-of-shape, 2-pack-a-day smoker of becoming a world-class athlete? What if I added that this same middle-aged gentleman got on a bike one day, for the first time since his youth and wobbled for 3 miles, just like a young kid learning to ride; and that the next day he was so sore that he said, "...I thought I would die from the pain. It was awful." NOW, what are the chances that he would become a world record holder in CYCLING, or even ever get back on a bike, for that matter?

Impossible odds or not, that's exactly what **Robert F. Beal** did. At 55, Robert retired as a successful businessman and after his first 3-mile foray on a bike decided that cycling would be a fun way to get back in shape. By age 72, he was an age-group world record holder and a training coach for the US Cycling Federation, preparing young athletes (3-time Tour De France champion Lance Armstrong being one of them) for world class and Olympic competition.

But, of course, it wasn't that easy. There were some hurdles along the way. For example, after six months of training Robert entered his first race — a 32 miler that he couldn't finish. He felt uncomfortable. He wondered whether a 55-year-old, fat, out-of-shape individual such as he belonged with these experienced bike racers. But early on he had made a good decision and joined a bike club. The support, advice, and camaraderie of the other members got him through these early weeks of self doubt and were just what he needed to keep going and become successful. Soon he was in his element and winning age-group awards.

It hasn't been just a bed of roses for Robert. He's had to train hard. At 72 he was putting in 300 miles a week on his bike, plus more hours in the gym working out. He's had two open-heart surgeries, and a little arthritis, a crash that broke 38 bones (yes, there apparently are 38 bones and more in our body) including his neck, and a fractured skull. You say, "I don't need any broken bones, thank you very much." And I say you can enjoy riding a bike, as recreation and a source of exercise, without skull fractures, broken bones and such. But if you are a highly-competitive person like Robert is, when you careen down mountain roads at over 50 miles per hour and negotiate hairpin turns at "breakneck" speeds, pushing the envelope of safety in order to win a race or improve your personal best time, you sometimes have to take your lickings, so to speak.

Now concerning the heart problems, you may be wondering why someone who gets his exercise — and then some — would suffer from heart disease. Robert is obviously very competitive, disciplined, and goal oriented; and while exercise in general is very good for us, at the elite level at which Robert is competing, one can sometimes overtrain or push himself too far in an effort to reach a significant goal. In my opinion, Robert's competitive drive made him a champion, but it is also what made him sick. He didn't listen to his body; when it asked for rest, he may have given it exercise to the point that it couldn't recuperate and thus broke down. For example, one day he was racing up a hill when he fell off his bike; he didn't know it, but it was a heart attack. The very next day, even though he felt terrible, he entered and finished a race to win a cycling title — then he went and had heart surgery. Robert, the champion, would probably argue that if it weren't for the cycling he would have died years ago. He might also add that it has given him something to live for; that it gives life to his life.

If Robert can overcome a lifelong smoking habit, two open-heart surgeries, multiple broken bones, and a little arthritis to become a champion cyclist in his sixties and seventies, riding 300 miles a week, then maybe we have little excuse not to take regular multi-mile walks, jogs, or bike rides just for the fun and restorative powers of it. Or maybe we can enter some competitions, as long as we listen to our body and heed its requests.

Permission to use quote from It's Never Too Late! given by Breakaway Books (BreakAwayBooks.com)

What Makes Grandma Run?

At 56, **Lucille Singleton** was taking care of an older lady when the woman's granddaughter, a runner, would come to visit. Their conversations reminded Lucille of how much she had loved to run as a child, not in organized competitions, but just racing friends in childhood play. Having spent most of her life doing for others as a child-care domestic, a housekeeper/cleaner, or a caregiver for the elderly, to support her children and such, she thought it was about time to do something for herself.

She joined the New York Runners' Club and started running. Afraid of coming in last, she would only run by herself (not in races). True to her nature, meanwhile, she, volunteeered to help at NYRC races — which she has now done for 19 years. During these years as a volunteer, she would, in her private life, get up at 3:30 every morning to run four solitary miles up 8th Avenue in Harlem. One of the races she would help with, year after year, was the New York City Marathon, giving out racing numbers, T-shirts, and the like. Seeing the excitement of the runners, she finally bit the bullet and entered her first race, a 3-miler, at age 67. Once she got that first race out of the way, she was on her way to racing 3-milers on a regular basis, often winning her age group, taking home trophies and ribbons, and very importantly to her — not finishing last.

At age 70, she was not ready to retire, but she did decide that she needed a new line of work. She ventured into, of all things, construction work. She continues to this day, doing carpentry work and plumbing as a New York City construction worker.

At age 75, Lucille finally got up the nerve to run her first marathon, but not just any marathon: one of the world's premier races, The New York City Marathon. With the support of all the myriad of friends and acquaintances she had made as a NYC marathon volunteer, over the years, she made it to the finish line with endless cheers, words of encouragement, AND HUGS along the way. Lucille later said that, "Crossing the finish line was the best moment of my entire life." Oh yes, and she didn't come in last!

If Lucille can muster up the courage to run her first marathon at age 75 and get up each morning at 3:30 to run in the dark, empty streets of Harlem, then maybe we can get a dog and take him for long, daily walks or we can take on a new, exciting challenge, such as ....

Permission for quote from It's Never Too Late! given by Breakaway Books — The Literary Sports Publisher

Strong Women Go Places And Do Things

In her highly recommended book, *Strong Women Stay Young,* author and renowned researcher at Tufts University Center on Aging, Miriam E. Nelson, Ph.D., tells of the tales of countless women who have benefitted from strength training. This is the story of one such woman, whom we'll call Granny (not her real name - who'd name their kid Granny? Not me).

Granny, a participant in one of Nelson's studies, continued to strength train after the year-long study concluded and also added 3-mile power walks to her weekly routine. Her fitness routine has so transformed her that her new-found youthfulness is apparent; it is so obvious that even her children's friends ask how she stays so healthy and looks so young.

With the restoration of her strength and energy, Granny was able to go on a family vacation that included whitewater rafting and horseback riding. The next summer she found herself parasailing in Hawaii, enjoying the beautiful view of Maui from several hundred feet up. The following summer she returned to Hawaii with her family to surf and ride the waves. Finally, she competed in the Senior Olympics and won a silver medal. That was a couple of years ago, so who knows what daring adventures she's had since then. Oh, I forgot to mention that Granny is the mother of 11 children, grandmother to 17, and 71 years young. She used to get depressed thinking she wouldn't be around to see her grandchildren grow up; now she thinks she may, after all.

The World Is His Stage

In his early adult years, **John Keston** sang and acted on stage and screen. In his mid fifties, running on tracks also became part of his "stage."

John had stayed in shape all his adult life, at a svelte 6 foot, 148 pounds, by playing squash and the like to be ready for whatever role came his way. In his fifties, the Brit, (now an

American citizen) was introduced to running. In his first race, at 55, he won his age-group in a 10K (6.2 miles). By age 63, he was a top-notch runner, turning in a 37:42 10K. Not only had he improved greatly, but his score would be good for a runner in his thirties.

In his sixties, John consistently ran marathons in sub-3-hour times; he is the oldest person to run a marathon in under 3 hours, having run a 2:58:32 just weeks before his seventieth birthday. He held the 70-74 age-group world record for 5 years with a 3:00:58 marathon, run in 1996; Ed Whitlock edged him off the record books in 2001 with a time of 3:00:24.

Unlike many runners who specialize in only "short" or "long" races, John excels at a variety of distances, as shown by his world record performance in 1995 when he ran a 5:34 mile at age 69. That is a score few 20-year-old runners will ever achieve.

At age 72, John was running more than 60 miles per week toward breaking world age-group records. But by 75, he was *down* to 45 to 55 miles due to a couple of serious injuries to his hip and ankle.

Having overcome his injuries, in 2001, at age 76, John renewed his assault on the record books with several age-group records, including: a 6:27 mile, a 41:59 10K, and a 3:22:59 marathon (the oldest runner ever to break 3:30). Here are three secrets to his return to top running form.

1. He now regularly allows 72 hours between runs for full recovery and to maintain muscle mass. This keeps him "feeling fresh" to enjoy his usual runs of two hours/15 miles at an 8 minute per mile pace, with some 7:00 to 7:15-minute miles in the middle. That's about 30 to 40 miles per week, including weekend races.
2. On "days off," he walks 2 to 4 miles, twice a day, to help with muscle recovery and weight control.
3. While others his age are stuck inside glued to their recliners, John is *getting more joy than ever* from his long, logging-trail runs.

Some 70-year-olds are in nursing homes, a burden on their children and grandchildren. Others, like John Keston are still pursuing their dreams and living life to its fullest. If John can set marathon records in his seventies, recording times that few adults of *any age* could run, then we can get up and get moving so that our arthritis or ... doesn't cripple us and make us dependent on others.

Speed Thrills

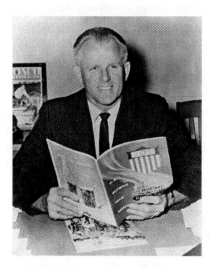

In 1941, in his mid-twenties, **Payton Jordan** set a world record in the 100-yard sprint with a blistering time of 9.4 seconds. Thirty years later, in 1972, at the age of 55, Payton came out of retirement to set a new age-group world record of 11.6 seconds for the 100-meter event; but, he didn't stop there. For most of the next 27 years he set age-group records in the 100 and 200-meter runs — the last being set at age 82. Although his speed has diminished *slightly* through the years, at age 74, for example, he was able to beat his world record from 7 years earlier, improving from 13 flat to 12.91.

People are amazed to find that in his mid-seventies he was still fast enough to beat all the students in a typical high school, with the exception of the best sprinters. How did Payton maintain such phenomenal speed through the years?

Payton was a head track-and-field coach for 40 years. Among other schools, he coached at Stanford University in California and was the head track coach for one of the U.S.A.'s best Olympic teams ever — the 1968 United States Mexico City team. Through the years, he kept himself in top shape so he could *show* his athletes what to do and to *lead by example.* This is one of the reasons why in 2000 he received the very prestigious Dwight D. Eisenhower Fitness Award. Recipients in previous years were former President George Bush and Arnold Schwarzenegger. Because of his high fitness level, he could have competed during his early-coaching years, but chose not to until age 55 partly because there wasn't a master's running program (competitions for ages 40 and older) until the early 1970s.

Before we delve into the secrets to Payton's retaining, decade after decade, so much of his astounding speed, let's learn a little more about the man, Payton Jordan. Payton is very generous with his time and likes to see others get into fitness and sports and to succeed. If he knew you personally, he would undoubtedly do everything he could to encourage you in any way he could. He might tell you, "Fear is our greatest enemy and desire is our greatest weapon." So if you are afraid to lift weights, for example, because of a concern for getting hurt or you are reluctant to enter athletics at your age, because you think you will look silly or finish last, then you've lost anyway. For one thing, you will have lost the opportunity to experience the wonderful feeling of "invigoration that comes from a good healthy workout." You will have missed out on the "joy of putting your capacity against someone else's and sharing the excitement and challenge together."

According to Jordan's philosophy of life, what makes a champion or allows the successful accomplishment of a goal is:

1. Commitment and goal setting
2. Discipline
3. A strong work ethic
4. Ability to appreciate and give credit to others

These are some of the attributes that are at the heart of Payton's becoming and staying one of the world's fastest men, generation after generation. These, plus family support and good genes, he would tell you. Finally, Payton would get around to letting you know that you shouldn't "...be afraid to dream big dreams. But don't daydream. Use your dreams to put yourself in motion and make things happen. Dreams and goals can be set high, but discipline must be high also. And that's where things break down."

These are words to live by, *my interpretation of Payton's philosophy and what his message to you would be, as ascertained from news clippings and other archival materials that Payton so graciously sent to me. The quotes were from these newspaper articles.*

If Payton can have dreams and goals to set world records in his seventies and eighties in a young man's sport, such as sprinting, then we can have a goal to hike the Swiss Alps or _____ and commit to it!

Stiff Is, As Stiff Doesn't

Most of us think that getting stiff and achy is a natural part of getting older. In actuality, aches and pains and losing one's flexibility, so often associated with aging, are mostly the result of inactivity and limiting thinking. **June Tatro** says it this way, "Age is not so much by the calendar, as it is by the way we believe and live; and loss [flexibility, balance, strength and endurance] is due to inactivity and is recoverable at any age."

June is living proof that she knows what she is talking about. At 87, she is a fitness instructor (a "physical conditionist") and still performs occasionally with her daughter as an *amateur* contortionist (she has even performed on *Oprah*) doing full splits, contorted handstands, and various positions I won't even attempt to describe here. June would have you know that you just don't suddenly decide to try to twist your body like a pretzel. Her fitness and skills as a contortionist are the result of taking care of herself through the years. Also, she wants me to explain that her profession does not have to be viewed as grotesque, with a side-show aura, but rather that it can be a beautiful, well respected artform as it is in Europe.

June has not acquired her agile fitness by running endless laps or weightlifting in a gym. Rather, she chooses to combine her "workouts" with everyday life. For example, she stands on her toes while talking on the phone; parks in distant corners of the parking lot and walks to the store; does deep breathing, and stress reduction exercises while sitting; and frequently ballroom dances with her husband.

June teaches fitness classes at the Escondido Adult School, where her students' average ages are in the seventies and eighties, with some nineties sprinkled in, including a couple of 95-year-olds. June is a teacher at heart and would love nothing more than to share her insights on healthy aging with you. From her voice on the phone, you can tell she is excited about life and loves her students and helping them reach their highest potential. Nothing excites her more than taking a client who doctors have proclaimed would never walk again and getting him or her up and walking and even ballroom dancing.

June has so much to tell us that she needs her own book. Here is just a sampling of her wisdom and knowledge (some of which she has shared on the Oprah Show and elsewhere).

1. **It is very important to warm up before attempting to stretch..** For example: Sit in a chair. Straighten the head and neck, as if you were a marionette with a string attached to your head being pulled straight up (the rest of your body will naturally follow and come into alignment). Silently count to 5 as a deep breath is taken in. Hold the breath, as you squeeze tight every muscle in your body, even squinting the eyes and gritting the teeth as hard as you can, while counting silently to 10. Then slowly breath out through pursed lips while counting silently to 10 again and relax all the muscles completely. Repeat this whole process 2 more times.

2. **Exercisers have fewer aches and pains than non-exercisers.**

3. **Poor posture can cause us to lose up to 30% of our oxygen consumption.**

4. **A good diet is very important — like fuel in a car.** In order of priority, eat vegetables, fruit, whole grains, low-fat dairy, fish, meats, fats and oils, and only an occasional sweet (junk food).

5. **Practice deep breathing anytime, anywhere throughout each day.**

6. **Concentrating on the exciting things about life is beneficial; too many people concentrate on health problems.**

If incorporating these simple little techniques and attitudes into June's life has helped make her this fit and excited about life, then we can make some of these techniques a part of our everyday life, too, so that the second half of our life can be *better* than the first.

Turning Excuses Into Records

What's our excuse for not getting the exhilerating, life-giving exercise our body/mind needs and craves? Too busy? Too tired? Too sick? Afraid we'll get hurt? Don't know what to do or how to do it? Too old? Too bad!

Here are some folks, just like you and me, who have turned excuses into reasons to get moving:

Let's start with **Evelyn Tucci.** At 82, her excuse could be that she is just getting too old to play golf; she might even twist something swinging those clubs at her age and injure herself, seriously. Instead, she plays golf for fun and to stay in shape and she stays in shape to play and enjoy golfing.

Evelyn and a friend entered a best-ball member/guest tournament at the Crystal Lake Country Club in Pompano, Florida. Lo and behold, she had the thrill of her life when she hit a hole-in-one on the par 3, 112 yard, No. 2 hole. But she wasn't through; just 3 holes later she shot her second ace. To cap it off, she and her partner, a Carin West, won the tournament with a handicapped score of fifty-five. Just because she's "too old" to golf didn't stop her from having one of the greatest days of her life and making the evening news across the country and the world.

While many of his peers snoozed in front of the TV, **David Clark,** 75, set sail to circumnavigate the world. That was in 1999. Two years later, he arrived back home in Fort Lauderdale, Florida, the oldest person to ever sail around the world solo (that is, by himself, if you don't count his dog, Mickey). To reach his goal, he had to withstand a week-long storm off the coast of Australia, with gale-force winds of 60 to 70 mph, during which he survived by "two-fisted holding on for a solid week." He also overcame his first boat, a 42-footer named Mollie Milar, taking on water in treacherous seas and sinking two days out of Cape Town, South Africa. David had the adventure of a lifetime, at an age when many have given up on life.

Then there is San Diego's **Tom Lane.** Tom is over 100 (yes, that is years old!) and blind (from a 1986 run-in with glaucoma), two excuses many of us would give for hanging up our swimming trunks and calling it a life. Tom saw it differently. He looked forward to swimming in meets once he had celebrated his 100th birthday so he could set new records in his next age-group, 100 to 104, that wouldn't be broken for a while due, in part, to the dearth of competitors in his age bracket. In 1995 he did just that, adding 5 world records (in the freestyle and backstroke 50 and 100 meter and yard sprints) to his already-large stash of world records and first-place finishes from previous years. Oh yes, Tom also likes to bowl, lift weights, golf, and throw the javelin — did I hear someone yell fore'!?

Gene Gerow could use the I'm-too-busy excuse to get out of taking his mother-in-law out for strolls during the weekends. You see, between work, family obligations, and his training for long-distance running races, Gene could seem to have too hectic a life for this little extracurricular activity. Instead, Gene, 56, pushes his 85-year-old, wheel-chair-bound mother-in-law, Blanche McNutt, for 5 miles at a 10-minute-per-mile pace. He enjoys a good relationship with Blanche, they have a good time together, *AND he gets in an extra workout.* Gene is a 1:45 half-marathoner (which averages out to sustaining about an 8:05/mile pace for 13.1 miles) and a nice-guy-in-law.

Just a youngster, at 46, **Jan Fuller** could use multiple sclerosis (whose symptoms she began noticing 7 years ago in 1995) as her excuse. Instead, she runs 6 miles three days a week before heading off to her teaching responsibilities as a speech and language therapist. As of 2000, she had run the Boston Marathon 6 consecutive years and was looking to run it again in 2001. Astonishingly, she ran a Boston Marathon qualifying time of 3:54 in 1999 (the other years she qualified and ran as a member of the Marathon Strides Against Multiple Sclerosis Team).

I'd be remiss if I didn't include *Ironmen* **Dick Hoyt and his son, Ricky,** in this group. Ricky, a college-educated young man who happens to be quadriplegic (for all intents and purposes) due to mutliple sclerosis, wanted to "do" the Hawaiian Ironman Triathlon. His father would have to "carry" him the whole way using his 59-year-old body to accomplish this astounding feat. Looking at the prospect of dragging his son on a raft as he swam the 2.4 miles of ocean; then immediately biking the rugged 112 miles with Ricky on a handlebar seat; and then running a full marathon while pushing him in a "stroller-racing-wheelchair," Dick could have said, "This race is too arduous to carry another human being, especially at my age."

On the other hand, Dick knew how much this would mean to Ricky. His love for his son drove him to train until he was, at 59, in the best shape of his life (as one look at his well-chiseled calf and forearm muscles could verify.).

Despite having to tow his son behind him on a raft, they made it through the swimming portion of the Ironman. Next came the cycling, where their competitors rode the finest that twenty-first century technology had to offer, with their gazillion gears and ultra-light aluminum frames; Dick and Ricky's transportation was a rickety, "Model T" of a bike with no bells and whistles, just 2 wheels, 2 seats, and handlebars. As Dick struggled to keep moving on this "antique" bike (piece of junk would be more like it), they slowed to a crawl. Eventually, the bike clanged and wobbled to a standstill and could go no more. Ricky was asked if he wanted to continue under the circumstances. He stated emphatically that he did and so they waited to have the bike repaired and then peddled into the night. Seventeen hours after the start of the race they completed the marathon run portion to the cheers of the crowd and the glare of the finish-line lights, as Ricky raised his arms triumphantly. Father and son savored the sensation of accomplishing that which few of us mere mortals would have dreamed possible. Sweet victory was *theirs* to savor.

Dick and Ricky have also enjoyed together the challenge of other races, including 21 years of running the Boston Marathon. A more recent race was the 2001 Boston classic, where Dick, now in his sixties, pushed Ricky the 26.2 miles to an enviable 3:19:04 finishing time. That time would be impressive for most 30-year-old marathoners even sans "wheelchairs" to push up Hearbreak Hill.

What is our excuse? What is our excuse, this time? One cannot put a price tag on the utter joy that comes from doing that which others deem impossible. If these ordinary individuals (Evelyn, David, Tom, Gene, Jan, Dick, and Ricky can

81

turn excuses into reasons, then maybe, just maybe, we can, too!

Last One In the Pool

Many of us think, even in our fifties, that to take up something new, such as a sport, or to renew our participation in an activity we enjoyed and/or excelled in as a young person is out of the question and puts our sanity in doubt. These National and World Champion swimmers you are about to meet are glad they didn't subscribe to such limiting thinking, and so are we.

Due to the United States Masters Swimming Program, they have been able to recommit to their aquatic passion and start competing again in swimming meets in their 60s, 70s and even 80s. These meets are open to swimmers from the age of 25 to 100 and beyond, in 5-year age groupings to give all competitors a level playing field (or should we say swimming pool?). There are local competitions around the country; National meets from Houston to Orlando; and World Championships from Rio deJaneiro to Tokyo to Brisbane, Australia to Sheffield, England.

Here are some senior athletes who, because they dared to try something "new," have enjoyed the accolades, medals, camaraderie, travel, and excitement that these competitions make possible.

Imagine first learning to swim when in your sixties, entering your first swim meet at age 70, and at age 80 breaking, by more than a full second, a 5-year-old 1,000-meter backstroke world record. That is exactly what **Sally Scott** of Miami has done. A life-long dancer, she also began competitive ballroom dancing at age 70. Sally has even danced the Tango at Madison Square Garden in New York City. From age 85 to 88, this late bloomer totaled 26 gold medal swims.

What's Sally's secret? She would swim 3,000 yards a day during her two-hour, 5-days-a-week workouts with a high school team near her home. She's also had a good diet, having been a vegetarian most of her life, eating huge quantities of raw fruits and vegetables.

Jean Durston took up swimming in her late fifties, after a serious illness, when her doctor suggested *some* aquatic exercise and therapy. A year later she started competing. Her first meet "... was traumatic," she recalled. "I drank a lot of pool water." About twenty-five years later she owned 14 world records. At 85, she swam the 200-meter butterfly in a world record 5:49.75 (an exhausting stroke that most of us couldn't swim for one length of the pool, never mind more than twice the length of a football field). She also received the David Yorzyk Memorial Award for a 400-yard, individual medley race at the Short Course National Championships where she broke the existing national record by more than 2 minutes.

Ann Bauscher was an All-American in numerous Masters events in almost every year from 1978 to 1998. In 1989, she was selected for the USMS Masters Swimming All-Star Team. This is an exceptional honor because only one male or female per age-group is selected out of 30,000 Masters swimmers. Ann returned home from Nationals each year from 1984 to 1990 with 4 gold medals. Yet, believe it or not, she didn't step into a swimming pool until she was 60 years old!

Unlike the others, **Peter Jurczyk** started swimming when he was five and won his first competition at seven. However, as an adult, life as a drill press operator and manufacturing engineer took him away from swimming competitions. Then in 1975, at the age of 69, he took the plunge back into competitive swimming. At age 91, in 1997, he was training 3 or 4 times a week, swimming a mile almost every time he hit the water; and he held 9 or 10 world records. Lest you think these world records are easy to get, you should know that at the Sixth World Masters Swimming Championships in England, where Peter won 8 medals, there were about 4,650 swimmers, age 25 and up, from 48 countries.

An Olympic champion in 1920 at age 14, **Aileen Riggin Soule** returned to competitive swimming in the mid-1980's at the youthful age of 80. By age 90, she was a Masters world champion with 5 world records and 11 national titles in the 90-to-94 age-group. Aileen, like Peter, would train by doing one nonstop mile per training session, three times a week.

If Sally, Jean, Anna, Peter, and Aileen can jump in with both feet at well past 50, then maybe we can find something new and exciting that we would enjoy doing — maybe swimming, maybe something else. Perhaps we were premature, by 20 or 30 years, in giving up a sport or other activity that gave us great joy and a sense of accomplishment. Maybe we could enjoy it again.

Sink Or Swim

Let's see if this next group of master swimmers will release any of their secrets to vibrant longevity — their being fitter after 50.

On swim teams in high school and college, in the 1920's and 30's, **Dave Malbrough** didn't return to competitive swimming until 1976, when he was near retirement at age 63. At his first national meet in 1976, he swam the 100-meter backstroke in 1:39.17; 17 years later, at age 80, his time was 1:45.81 - less than 7 seconds slower. At 85, he broke Tom K. Cureton's 12-year-old record in the 50-yard backstroke with a 46.81; he also claimed world champion Gus Langner's 500-yard freestyle mark, finishing in 9:55.12. How did he maintain such an impressive fitness and skill level?

Tom Cureton, a well-known fitness expert whose record as we just noted, Dave broke, became Dave's friend and mentor. Cureton, an early advocate of vitamin E (long before it became fashionable), got Dave on a supplement and nutrition program (including skim milk, for example). Dave felt that this, plus his training, helped slow down the aging process, allowing him to retain much of his swimming speed over the years.

At age 81, **Walt Pfeiffer** of Mission Viejo, CA, set twelve world records. He set these new marks in some tough swims, such as the 200-meter fly and the 400-meter individual medley, breaking the old records by an eye-popping 10, 20, and even 50 seconds. When Walt reached the 85-to-89 age-group in 1998 and 1999, he set 11 more world records, including an impressive 9:31.75 in the 400 individual medley. His record-producing training consisted of swims of about 2,000 yards (that's *20 lengths of a football field*, to put it in perspective) 3 or 4 times per week. He, also, enjoyed working out with his wife, Annetta, and others "his age" or thereabouts.

Mildred Anderson learned to swim when she was 14 and entered her first competition at 18. She and her husband, Ham, got into Masters swimming after age 50. Mildred did okay, being designated an All-American 9 times during the 1970's and 1980's. She received the Ransom J. Arthur Award in 1978; this award is given each year to one male and one

84

female swimmer who has done the most to further the objectives of masters swimming (Ransom J. Arthur established the Masters Swimming Program in the U.S. to improve the health of adults through swimming).

Mildred has said that the masters swimming has given her a sense of achievement and that it was excellent therapy for her back (at the time, Mildred had experienced four significant injuries to her back and also had arthritis).

In 1997 and 98, at the ages of 80 and 81, **Aldo DaRosa** broke more than 80 regional, national, and world records. When he's not in training or competing, Dr. DaRosa is a professor of electrical engineering at Stanford University.

Dr. DaRosa's record-breaking performances are the result of swimming 6 or 7 days a week for about 2,200 yards per session. He thrives on the camaraderie of swimming on a team. Besides swimming, his training includes approximately one hour of stretching each day, some weight training, and he incorporates scheduled rest periods before big meets and distance swims.

After swimming competitively as a youth, **Lavelle Stoinoff** got back into swimming in her forties to lose weight. She did poorly in her first race at age 44 and used this "failure" as motivation. It must have worked, because the very next year she won at nationals. In 1998, now in her mid-sixties, Lavelle was recognized as Masters Swimmer of the Year — holding about 9 world records. She specializes in the longer, more grueling races, such as the 400, 800, 1500-meter freestyle and the 200, 500, 1650-yard freestyle.

Lavelle is a big believer in stretching and lifting weights. She also jumps rope and runs 2 miles on the days she's not lifting. I almost forgot her 6-days-a-week, supervised-swimming workouts in which she averages 4,000-plus yards per session. She watches her fat intake and eats well, too. I wonder what the secret to her success is?

Lavelle has had 2 rotator-cuff surgeries which have put her out of commission for long periods of time; so maybe she's overtraining. Perhaps the forced rest during rehab has helped her in the long-run.

G. Harold "Gus" Langner was a competitive swimmer all his life. He loved swimming. He was good enough in his youth to make it to the 1928 Olympics trials where he competed against "Buster" Crabbe (best known for playing Tarzan in the movies).

Gus did okay later on in his life in masters swimming. From age 80 to 94, he held, at one time or another, 185 world records and 329 national records. He began swimming again in the late 1950's just for the fitness benefits, after a 25-year layoff, and after President Eisenhower's heart attack started a national physical fitness movement; and then he entered Masters swimming in the 1970's.

According to Dr. Phil Whitten, author of *The Complete Book of Swimming,* at 91 Gus looked at least 25 years younger and had the strength and endurance of a man half his age. His specialty was the distance events, and he loved to compete; but also swam for the fun and the health of it. At 91, he could swim a mile in about 36 minutes (most of us would drown in about 5 minutes).

Gus, Dave, Mildred, Aldo, and Lavelle swam for the fitness benefits, the fun of competing, the carmaraderie at meets, the feelings of accomplishment, and as role models for the rest of us. They *loved* to swim, too!

So what is their secret? Is it the endless laps in the pool? Is it the stretching and strength training? Is it knowing when to schedule rest periods and breaks in training? Is it their diet and supplements? Is it their love of swimming? Yes, these all play a part in their success equation. However, the real secret to their success, what kept them coming back for more laps when they didn't feel like it, was the dream. The dream of new personal bests, gold medals, national titles, and world records. This is the impetus that caused them to do what they needed to do to be champions. And this action that evolves out of the imagination, the dreaming, is what made them so successful, so happy, and so much fitter after 50.

If these folks can benefit so greatly from dreaming (imagining) big dreams, then what can we dream that will motivate us? What would we love to do?

Life Begins At 58

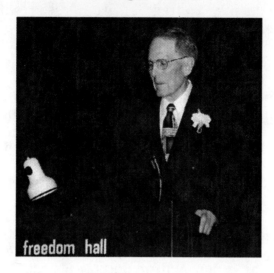

When **Warren Utes** took his army physical in 1941, he was a fit-and-trim 146 pounds. A smoker in his young adult years, he quit in his early thirties and began to put on weight. As with many of us, his poundage crept up steadily over the years until in his mid-fifties he found himself weighing in at 178 to 180. Although that put him 30 pounds overweight, he was still in relatively good shape.

Inspired by the Olympic competitions he witnessed on TV in the 1970's, at the age of 58 Warren decided to give running a try. He joined a running club, where he could learn from more experienced runners and benefit from being "pulled along" by the younger, stronger racers — so as to reach more of his potential. The new friends he made, the fun competing, and his early successes spurred him on to a successful career, to say the least.

Warren is now 80 and still going strong. What does he have to show for his 22-plus years of racing? Just a lot of good times and 69 or 70 (who can keep track) national age-group records in everything from the 800 meters to marathon distances and the honor of being elected to the USA Track and Field Masters Hall of Fame. Warren ran his last marathon, the Twin Cities Marathon, in an impressive 3:36:59, at age 78, when the only "mileage" many of his peers put in is the distance from their bed to the bathroom on their nightly sojurns. But that's not all. Thanks to his running and other good health habits, Warren is also blessed with excellent health (his blood tests and other readings from his regular check-ups are all in the normal range). While quite a few 80-year-olds are spending $2,000 per year and more for prescription medicines to keep them alive and out of pain, Warren takes no medication at all, unless you want to count the baby aspirin tablet he takes each day just to be on the safe side.

Now that he has turned 80, is Warren going to put his feet up and rest on his laurels? When I talked with him, he was hibernating during another Chicago-area winter of ice and snow and bitter-cold winds off the lake. During "hibernation," he was putting in 30 to 60 minutes a day on his treadmill while he eagerly awaited the Spring thaw and the return of good running weather. With the good weather, he was looking forward to getting out and running his 6.4 mile course in the woods behind his home and logging 20 or more miles each week, plus doing some speed work. In past years, he would routinely put in 50 miles per week, and 60 before a marathon. At one time he was doing 75 miles, but he found that that was too much for his body to endure without injuries.

In the Spring of 2001 Warren was looking forward to running in a team event in Southern Illinois, where 8 runners run a total of 80 miles (about 10 miles each in three 5K segments). He was also planning for a local 10K, where he could set some more age-group records. *Postscript: Since I wrote the above, Warren has indeed run in the team event (a sixth place), turned 81 (June, 2001), and run 14 more races — including a national age-group 5K record (pending) with an amazing 21:59.*

To keep his body healthy and fit so that he can race well and set new records, Warren sees to it that his body is well cared for. He tunes in to his body's signals so that he doesn't overtrain; and he warms up and stretches before each run. In the past, when he hasn't listened to his body and prepared properly for each outing, he's ended up too often with injuries in the form of sprained ankles, shin splints (75 miles/week), bursitis of the heel (wearing the same shoes run after run), and sciatica. He's scaled down his mileage to give his body the rest it needs for optimal recuperation after each exercise session.

Diet-wise Warren eats well, consuming more fruits and vegetables than anything else — frequently stir-frying with tofu and vegetables. He also watches the fat in his diet and drinks plenty of fluids. Supplements consist of a daily dose of vitamin E (400IU).

I asked Warren what he would like to tell you, our readers:

1. Keep moving; it is the healthy thing to do.
2. Run, play tennis, or whatever with younger folks; they pull you along and make you better.
3. Drink plenty of fluids — mostly water, but also drinks such as green tea.
4. Set little goals all the time. For example, make the decision to work out tomorrow for 30 minutes or to catch the runner in front of you during a workout run or a race.
5. Start with modest plans and build. Set reasonable goals; don't be too ambitious.
6. Persistence is the key. Run or exercise regularly — not in fits and starts or off and on again.
7. If you are the competitive type, design a well-structured workout plan to expand your limits and set new personal bests.

If Warren has this much vim and vigor at 81, while keeping the record-book statisticians extremely busy, then maybe we should take to heart what his life and wisdom have to tell us!

Only the Strong Shall Thrive

The main reason individuals slow down as they get older is because they typically lose about one-third of their muscle mass between the age of 35 and 80. Study after study has shown that strength training can reverse this trend in even the oldest and frailest.

Scientists at Ohio University found that 60 to 75-year-old men, who were put on just a 2-day-per-week, high-intensity weight training program, in a mere 16 weeks increased their strength by an average of up to 84 percent. Specifically, their strength gains averaged 50 percent for their leg extensions, 72 percent for leg presses, 84 percent for half squats. Likewise, their endurance improved, as shown on treadmill tests.

89

Miriam E. Nelson, Ph.D., a researcher on aging at Tufts University, reports on a study of the effects of strength training on postmenopausal women. Twenty of the women lifted weights two times per week; the other twenty were the non-exercising control group. According to Dr. Nelson, the strength-training group made small, but significant, gains in bone density, while the controls lost bone density, as expected. Also, the strength scores for the strength trainers rose to levels more often associated with 30 and 40-year-olds. In essence, after just one year of training, their bodies were biologically 15 to 20 years younger.

William Evans and Maria Fiatarone, M.D., also of the Tufts University Center on Aging, decided to see what benefits strength training would have for the weakest and frailest among us. They took ten typical nursing-home residents, four men and six women volunteers, ages 86 to 96, and put them on a strength-training program. All of them had at least two serious chronic diseases, such as heart disease, osteoporosis, and diabetes; most of them relied on canes and walkers to get around. The startling results of the eight-week study were published in JAMA (the Journal of the American Medical Association) in 1990. Their strength had increased an average of 175 percent and their balance and walking scores were up 48 percent. This inspired larger clinical studies at Tufts and elsewhere that verified the benefits of strength training in our older population.

But enough with the faceless statistics; let's look at how strength training has transformed the lives of specific people. Here are two individuals who took Bill Phillips' Body For Life Challenge. In this million-dollar contest, participants see how much they can transform their bodies and lives through a program centered on strength training with a little bit of aerobics thrown in to balance out the program.

A motorcycle accident at age 72 forced **Daniel Weidner** to rebuild his body. The ex-Marine, retired social studies teacher, and part-time mountain climber decided he wasn't through living, so he took on the Body For Life Challenge. Due to the accident, his usually fit, 150-pound body was down to 143. Over several months of weight training, he added 15 pounds of muscle, to become a muscular 158 pounds. This included dropping his waist size from 34 to 32 inches; increasing his chest from 33 to 38 inches; and growing his biceps from 12 to 14.5 inches. What can a 72-year-old do with such a fit body? How about a 3,000-mile bike ride from New Jersey to California (that is the plan) and maybe a return to the mountain climbing he loves?

Jeffry Life, M.D., Ph.D., at age 60, had a total cholesterol count of 248, and knowing the dangers of high cholesterol, was considering starting cholesterol-lowering medication. Dr. Life had tried different methods to get it down, including following the low-fat, low-protein, high carbohydrate diet recommended by cardiologists and nutritionists. Knowing that he would probably have to take a cholesterol-lowering drug for the rest of his life, and being aware of the potential negative side-effects, he decided, instead, to try strength training (specifically, the Body For Life Challenge, with its special diet for gaining muscle).

The results were nothing short of phenomenal; he won the contest, reducing his percentage of bodyfat from 25% to 8.5 %, lowering his total cholesterol to a healthy 157 (decreasing his LDL "bad" cholesterol by 53%) and adding 14 pounds of muscle to his 60-year-old frame. Not bad for about 12 weeks of a special program of strength training, aerobics, and a special strength-building/fat-burning diet. And, of course, there was no need for the medication.

John W. Rowe, M.D. and Robert L. Kahn, Ph.D., in their book, *Successful Aging,* profile a senior citizen they just call **Edward**. According to them, Edward had hardly exercised a day in his whole life until he was 86, when he became a participant in a MacArthur Foundation study of the effects of weight training on the elderly. Despite living with peripheral neuropathy, a condition that robs the legs of a great deal of feeling, Edward completed the study, which included lifting weights three times per week. He found it so rewarding that five years after the study concluded, at age 91, he was still lifting religiously. Edward claims that the strength training helps his walking and makes him feel, sleep, and eat better. He even had to buy a new suit because his chest had gotten bigger, even though he weighed the same.

Women have had similar, miraculous life-enriching run-ins with weight training. Dr. Miriam Nelson's website, www.StrongWomen.com, and her book, *Strong Women Stay*

Young, are filled with examples of women 50 and older who sing the praises of strength training. One such individual is a lady named **Jeanne** who was diagnosed with osteopenia at age 66. This greatly perplexed her since, at the time, she was taking aerobics class three times per week and walking almost an hour on most other days. After following Dr. Nelson's strength-building protocol for a year and a half, she reports that her bone density tests had shown an increase in her left hip and a very significant 7.1 percent improvement in her lumber spine area, putting her back in the normal range.

If a strength regimen is really this good and these folks (Jeffry, Daniel, Edward, and Jeanne) have gained so much from lifting, then what wonderful surprises await us when we take up strength training? Maybe we, too, can become 15 to 20 years younger — without all the complications of renting a time machine.

Surfing for Life

If something gives you great joy, then why give it up just because the dates on a calendar proclaim that you are ancient? This is the thinking of the pioneers of surfing who are still riding the waves every chance they get. The sport that has been synonymous with reckless, irresponsible youth is now being shared with septenarians, octogenarians, and even novenarians.

John H. "Doc" Ball, at 93, is the oldest living American surfer — still surfing! Doc, a professional photographer and dentist, also likes to skateboard when he's not riding a big wave.

Waikiki Beach's **Rabbit Kekai** still teaches surfing at 80. He also surfs almost every day and recently won a 40-and-over surfing competition.

When David Nolan, a writer interviewing Rabbit, mentioned that he would like to take surfing lessons some day, Rabbit put him on the spot to learn right then and there. With just 15 minutes of dry-land instruction and another 15 in the water, David, in his fifties (and self-professed to lack flexibility, good reflexes, and courage), was up and surfing — hanging ten for about 100 yards.

Peter Cole, a legendary big-wave surfer, continues to surf the giant waves, 10 to 20 footers, in Hawaii. At 70, he is probably the oldest surfer to do so.

The inventor of the catamaran, **Woody Brown,** at 88, still surfs every chance he gets, when he's not volunteering at the Adult Day Health Center in Maui. In his youth he split his time between surfing and flying gliders.

Men aren't the only ones enjoying a life-long love affair with the surf. Seventy-four-year-old **Eve Fletcher** represents the distaff side of senior surfers. Being a woman, Eve wasn't compelled to ride the *big* ones to show her macho-ness, so she could milk the smaller waves for all their thrills. Therefore, while the men have their best rides behind them, Eve doesn't have to scale back her rides. As recently as age 71, she caught one of her best waves, an 8-footer, at San Onofre.

Anona Napoleon, 59, and **Shay Bintliff, M.D.**, 62, are two more female surfers who have been riding for years, since the sixties.

If Doc, Rabbit, Peter, Woody, Eve, Anona, and Shay are not too old to surf and if David Noland can learn to surf in just minutes, at 54, then what could we do? What have you always wanted to do? Imagine what it would be like to do it now!

CHAPTER 4 MINDING YOUR OWN BUSINESS

The exercises in this chapter will not have us huffing and puffing and sweating profusely, because they are gentle mental techniques. These cerebral activities will prevent procrastination (unless, of course, we procrastinate in using them) and help us stick with our program to create a leaner, stronger, healthier and more radiant version of ourselves.

The Success Twins

The success twins, desire and belief, whom we met in chapters one and two, will make us fitter after 50 if they join together in a concerted effort. However, if we have the desire to be fit, but don't really believe that we can do it because we lack the time or energy; or if we think that individuals over 50 are doomed to a steady descent into a feeble, frail old age no matter what they do — then our desire will be for naught. When belief is lacking we will procrastinate because deep down we don't believe anything of any significance will come of our efforts; or we will start out like gangbusters trying to make up overnight for years of lifestyle mistakes, and as a result of overdoing get dicouraged by sore muscles, injury, illness or lack of immediate results, and quit or gradually drift away from our fitness-recapturing program.

On the other hand, if belief is strong but desire is weak, then we won't have the interest needed to do anything about the shape we are in. Belief and desire must work hand in hand for us to get the tangible, rewarding results we would like and that James Hill and Helen Klein, from chapters 2 and 3, enjoy. The techniques in this chapter will strengthen our desire and belief and get them to work in tandem.

We all have a self-image of ourselves. We see ourselves as engineers, mothers, gardeners, stamp collectors, basketball fans, retired folks, cat lovers, etc. We also see ourselves as young, middle-aged, or old; skinny, fat, or getting fatter all the time; one who can eat anything and never put on a pound or one who can just look at food and put on weight; flexible and feeling good or stiff and arthritic; healthy and robust or heart-diseased; tired and burned out or in love with life; un-athletic, a former jock or athletic; old and sickly or fitter after 50.

These are our self-images. This is how we see ourselves. In order to make *lasting* changes, one must change his image of himself. As long as we see ourselves as fat or a little overweight, etc., we can lose 10 pounds, or even 20, on a diet and/or exercise progam and it will all (and maybe a little more) come right back to our hips and belly, where it belongs according to our view of ourself, because we haven't changed our mental self image — just the physical.

We identify ourselves by our self-image. It is who we are. Our self-image is like the thermostat in our home that regulates the temperature. When we lose too much weight, it "clicks off" to slow the metabolism and increase hunger to return us to our "proper"/normal weight (our inner vision of ourself). Likewise, when we gain too much weight it "clicks on" to burn the added fat and restore us to our accustomed weight and appearance. If our self-image is of one who is gaining weight then our thermostat (self-image) is constantly being reset to a higher reading. Unless we permanently change our thermostat setting (our self-image) to where we would like it, no amount of exercise or dieting will ever make any permanent, lasting change.

The mind and body will fight to preserve our image of ourself, this status quo, (e.g., old, fat, listless, etc.) because to do otherwise is annihilation of ourself as we know ourself to be. As long as we give our full attention to what we *are* (or currently perceive ourselves to be), then we can't become anything else, such as vibrant, energetic, passionate, and fitter after 50.

The Fitter-After-50 techniques that follow are our way to transform our self-image to something much more empowering, rewarding, and joyous. Without these mental techniques, we will most likely eat well, reduce our stress, and work out on a regular basis for a week, a month, or even a whole year and then gradually return to our comfort zone — our current vision of who we are — old and getting older; fat and getting fatter; etc. In this regard, according to sports psychologist William F. Morgan of the University of Wisconsin-Madison, 50 percent of those who start an exercise program quit within six to eight weeks and another 25 percent don't make it a whole year. Use these *FA50* techniques to avoid becoming just another dropout statistic.

If you like, really like, your present condition/self, then that is wonderful and you don't really need this book and its ideas. On the other hand, if you are tired of being sick and tired, overweight, out of shape, and/or looking and feeling "old," then together we can change your life drastically for a more joyous future.

Going to the Movies

As long as our focus is on our current condition (e.g., overweight, stressed out, tired and listless, out of shape, etc.), all we can get is more of the same. When we turn our attention instead to what we desire, then we can begin moving towards this new and improved us.

This life-changing technique draws its power from the fact that our mind doesn't differentiate between an actual event and a vividly imagined one. An example of this was shown in a segment of TV's Dateline news-magazine show. Two expectant mothers were taught how to use auto-hypnosis to control the pain of childbirth. One was new to giving birth and the other mother-to-be had had a "bad" (read that painful) experience the first time. The camera crew followed their progress through hours of labor and the actual birthing process. What we the viewers saw and were told was that both ladies had a pain-free, comfortable birthing experience from start to finish. If I hadn't seen it I wouldn't believe it either. The mind truly is the creator of our experience.

Another example is one we have all experienced firsthand and that is mistaking a dream for a real-life experience. It all seems so real until we awaken — heart racing, sweat dripping off of our brow — to realize that the nightmare scenario was just that, a nightmare.

To make your own fitness-enhancing movies, get into a comfortable, relaxed sitting position (or lying, if you promise you won't go to sleep). Close your eyes and take a deep breath and slowly let it out while feeling your body melt into your chair. Using as many of your senses as you can, imagine yourself the way you would like to be. For example, you are walking on the beach with your new sleek figure/physique. Pride wells up inside you as you experience the power and grace in each stride, the flat stomach, the people on the beach noticing how attractive you are. Hear a friend or family member telling you how great you look and know they really mean it. Hear the waves crashing on the beach, smell the sea breeze, feel the sand between your toes, notice the gentle warmth of the sun. The more vivid the scene and the more details you can experience, the better. Most importantly, get in touch with the positive feelings: the confidence, joy, goose-bumps, excitement, enthusiasm, peace, etc. The key is the positive feelings!

Or maybe you'd rather imagine/experience running your first marathon and the thrill of crossing the finish line with your friends and family there to greet you and cheer for you. How about picturing what it would be like to go to your high school reunion in your new body? Of course, it could be experiencing, in your mind, dancing the night away to your favorite tunes, in an elegant or "hip" wardrobe. Whatever your Oscar-winning "movie," the key ingredients are:

1. Go to your mental movie theater for the same reason you go to the movies at your local cinaplex - for the *entertainment* value. Your imagination should be a fun place to go and hang out. If you go there to try to manipulate the future, it won't work well because it will make you too aware of what you don't have. If we are unhappy where we are, we can't get anywhere else. We have to enjoy the journey, and our internal movie theater is part of that joyful journey to new circumstances — fitness after 50.
2. Go to the movies for two to five minutes twice a day. You can do more or less depending on your enjoyment level.
3. The more details, the more vivid, the better.
4. Emphasize and get in touch with your good/positive feelings.
5. Produce your movie in "first person" and present time. Experience the events as if they were real in your present time moment.

Remember, when we have something good in our life, we can give it our full attention, savor it, and appreciate it, and thereby set ourselves up for more of the same. When that in our life is not what we would like, we can Go To The Movies — our personally-produced ones in our imagination — and create/experience more of that which we would rather have.

Regular Emotional Check-Ups

Young children are excited, confident, enthusiastic, energetic, vibrant, and joyful (unless they are sick, ...). This is because the Life Force, God Force, Universal Energy, Universal Intelligence, whatever you choose to call it, is flowing freely and fully to and through them. This is the same energy or intelligence that created the world and causes the trillions upon trillions of cells in our body to work together to sustain life. When we die this Life Force or Soul withdraws from the body leaving an inanimate, lifeless pile of chemicals/molecules where just moments before there was a living, vibrant entity. Through the years between birth and death, we pick up disempowering mental baggage which we then proceed to lug around with us wherever we go. These negative, debilitating thoughts and beliefs limit the flow of Universal Intelligence to and through us and thus we lose the joy and enthusiasm for life that we had as a young child. These thoughts and beliefs gradually choke off more and more of this energy which created us and sustains us, until we finally die from a lack of this Life Force. We might compare this to the plumbing in our homes. When the pipes are new, they are wide open and the water flows through them freely and powerfully. But over the years more and more crud builds up on the inner walls and the water flow becomes more and more restricted until it is just a trickle or worse.

What are these disempowering thoughts and beliefs? One is that we deteriorate as we age. Another could be that "the world is going to hell in a handbasket." Worrying about our children, our finances, our health, our neighborhood, our schools, our society, etc. limits our joy — our Life Force.

Luckily, we have a guidance system that lets us know when we are restricting the flow of life-giving energy to us. It is called our emotions. Whenever we feel emotions, we are being guided or alerted to whether we are allowing Life Force to flow freely to and through us or whether we are choking it off. Negative emotions let us know we are heading right toward what we don't want. The reason we feel bad is because these negative feelings are the result of our cutting off, to some degree, the Life Force that would otherwise make us feel joyful, enthusiastic, courageous, confident, loved, and loving. Positive emotions tell us that in *the moment when we are feeling them* we are one with our True Self or Higher (infinite) Self, and this feels good.

Anytime we feel negative emotions, whether it is fear, anger, irritation, sadness, depression, guilt, jealousy, or some other variation of negativity, it is a wake-up call for us to change our thinking. Emotions are the result of how we think about or *perceive* a circumstance (or are an automatic neuro-association [e.g., a song reminds us of a lost love]). They are not the result of the actual event or circumstances themselves.

If someone cuts us off in traffic, it is not this event itself that causes the squeezing off of our Life Force, the negative emotion we feel; rather, it is our reaction to this circumstance and our thinking about it that makes us feel badly. We can think, "That idiot oughtn't be on the road!" and get madder and madder as we continue to focus on the other person's poor driving habits. As a result of this line of thinking, our blood pressure rises dangerously high and we get stressed out. Our muscles tighten and tense in preparation for a fight or flight, neither of which usually happens. Therefore, we hold on to the tension, which can result in a tension headache or achy, tense neck, shoulder, and back muscles. If we dwell on this relatively innocuous and minor event long enough (along with other daily irritations), we can even get sick or do something stupid and become the other idiot on the nightly news with Tom, Dan and Peter. On the other hand, we can always choose a thought that feels better. We can give the other driver the benefit of the doubt. We can think, "Well, maybe his pet boa constrictor just died and his mind is not on his driving," and then let it go. Or we could surmise that, "Maybe his shorts are too tight" and move on. Or we could thank him for being such a poor driver because in comparison he makes us look like Dale Jarrett, the race-car driver. Without the likes of him, *we'd* be the one others would say, "That moron shouldn't be allowed on the road!"

When you feel negative emotions, know that you are restricting the flow of Life Force that keeps us biologically young. Arnold Fox, M.D., a specialist in cardiology and a commissioner on the California State Board of Quality says, "...every thought in our head — positive or negative — affects our internal biochemistry." Nevertheless, keep in mind that negative emotions are good in that they let us know unequivocally when we are heading away from being fitter after 50. It's only when we continually dwell on thoughts that result in negative emotions that we start to do damage to our body and mind. Prolonged exposure to destructive thoughts (apparent by our emotions) depresses the immune system and otherwise limits the Life Force necessary to keep the body/mind system healthy and fit. For example, when scientists at Carnegie-Mellon University injected cold viruses into volunteers, they found that their susceptibility to catching a cold was directly correlated with the stress the subjects were feeling. This famous study, published in the New England Journal of Medicine in 1991, shows the effects of our negative thoughts and emotions on our well-being.

In another study reported in the Journal of American Geriatrics, subjects ages 63 to 82 played a computer game in which words were flashed on the screen subliminally. One group was subjected to "negative" words: "senile," "dependent," and "diseased." The other group was exposed to "positive" words: "accomplished," "astute," and "wise." Subsequently, there was no change in the walking speed of those who saw the "negative" words, but the participants who witnessed the "positive" words increased their walking pace by 9 percent.

Finally, Thomas P. Sculco, M.D., director of orthopedic surgery at the Hospital for Special Surgery in New York, who has performed thousands of hip replacements, says that "stress affects wound healing ... and recovery." That is, individuals who focus their thoughts on what they fear could happen (causing stress) heal slowly.

Regular Emotional Check-Ups means monitoring your feelings throughout the day. When you find negative emotions, whether they be just irritations or a slight sense of being stressed or whether they are full-blown raging anger, sorrow or guilt, take a minute to get in touch with the thoughts that are causing this emotion and *then choose a thought that feels better.* If you don't have time to deal with it then and there, make a mental note (or jot it down on a piece of paper, ...) to look at it later when you have a minute. Little upsets can be dealt with quickly and easily by choosing on the spot a thought that feels better. Big problems will take more time; but, by gradually softening your thoughts on the matter, over time, they too can be dealt with.

Remember, as a rule, little children are happy in the moment — vibrant and confident — because they don't dwell on what happened last week, yesterday, or even five minutes ago. Thus, they laugh, giggle, and smile frequently and love us unconditionally. They have much to teach us about LIFE. Smile, laugh, giggle, and love more often. Check your emotions often and choose thoughts that make you feel better, and you will be well on your way to being fitter after 50.

Make A "Whys" List

This exercise strengthens our desire to be fitter. After the novelty of starting an exercise program, improving our diet, or initiating a stress-reduction plan has worn off, we need a strong desire to be fit and healthy to keep us going. This technique will keep us getting out of that warm bed day after day to work out or keep us choosing that extra helping of broccoli over the rich, tempting dessert.

Most of us start by focusing on *how* to get fit, rather than the *why* to get fit. We overlook the fact that when the *why* is all-consuming (and the belief is unwavering), then the how will almost take care of itself. With the *why* front and center, the how will usually fall into our lap; we will be guided to it.

Focusing on the *why* keeps us in the creative mode — the creation of our new body. The *how* mode deals with managing our fitness, but can quickly turn into doubt. As Helen Klein told us in the last chapter, "...When doubt moves in your goal is given low priority in your mind." *How* thinking often deteriorates into:

How in the world am I going to get fitter after 50?

How can I possibly exercise enough to make a difference?

How can I be expected to ...?

How indeed?

To make a "Whys"list:

1. Mentally make a list of reasons why you want to get fit and number them. For example:

1) So I can have the energy to enjoy my precious family at the end of a long day.
2) So I can be a role model for my loved ones to take care of themselves.
3) So that I can wow them at my next reunion.
4) So I can be independent all my days.

2. Before you start, decide how many *why's* you are going to state — 5, 10, 20, or ...

3. As you state each reason, *feel* the good emotions that go with it.

4. Do this exercise at least once in writing and many times "orally" over the course of the first two months of your makeover, preferably at least once daily.

5. Keep adding to the number of reasons and get more precise and detailed about each reason.

6. Be spontaneous. In other words, don't be locked in to memorizing any set order or set of reasons. Feel free to add, drop, and modify your *why's*.

7. You can go through your list while primping in front of the mirror in the morning, while driving, before meals, right before bed, ...

Remember, the more intense your desire, the more drawn you will be to working out or eating well when challenged with a strong reason to skip a workout or succumb to that craving for fudge. Making good choices is easy when you have an intense desire to be fitter after 50.

The Appreciation Game

We live in a Universe created and held together by the fact that like attracts like. Solid is attracted to other solids; liquid to liquids; and gas to gases. Therefore, when a rock is dropped into a lake it falls to or is attracted by the the other solid matter at the bottom of the lake. Gases released by the Earth travel unerringly up through the ocean to mingle with the other gases in our atmosphere. Heart cells congregate with other heart cells to form the organ we know as the heart and they all work in tandem to pump blood. The heart cell never gets fed up with his job and migrates to become a liver or kidney cell. The bones of an Egyptian mummy can be wrapped in a burial cloth for thousands of years and yet, not a single molecule of those bones will have switched allegiance to become the cloth. A man and a woman are attracted to each other because of their similar interests (because of how they are alike), even if it is only the sex (their differences don't attract — they only complement one another).

When we think about a subject we tend to attract similar thoughts. For example, if we ruminate about how someone has mistreated us, we attract other similar thoughts of how this person and other individuals have done us wrong in other ways.

In **The Appreciation Game** the challenge is to see how many things we can appreciate about our body/mind. By doing this, we find more and more to appreciate (or love) about ourselves. Heart-felt gratitude is one of the most empowering positive emotions known to man. As such, it allows more and more of the Life Force that created us and maintains our well-being. These empowering thoughts will strengthen the immune system, improve digestion, build muscle, repair damaged cells, and otherwise create optimal well-being — one who thrives, not just survives. Like attracts like, appreciative thoughts create a body/mind that we can truly appreciate.

When we appreciate ourself (read that, love), we tend to take better care of ourself. Taking better care of ourself, we get in better shape. When we are fit and healthy we have more to appreciate. This being the case, we treat ourself well so as not to do harm to this self that is serving us so well. And so the cycle to a fitter, healthier us goes on and on, round and round. As it is with the fine motor car that we keep well fueled, lubricated, and serviced to give us endless, trouble-free, pleasurable driving miles, so too it is with our body/mind.

Here are some rules for playing the Appreciation Game:

1. Decide on how many aspects of yourself you are going to enumerate and feel appreciation for. For example, 10, 20, 50, 100, ...).
2. State the number "1" (silently or out loud) and picture a giant, colorful numeral number one in your mind's eye.
3. Think of something for which you are *really* grateful, such as your eyesight, skin, liver, fingernails, blood pressure, ... You may have some affliction; perhaps it is heart disease or

103

arthritis. But for each problem, there are always countless other ways our body works well. You can always be thankful for the improvement in a bodily function, too.

4. State the number "2" and continue as with number "1" (step or rule 2.)
5. These mental gymnastics can be performed while resting, driving, walking, running, ...
6. *Feel* a real sense of appreciation or thankfulness with each enumerated item.
7. This can be enjoyed with a partner, by taking turns telling each other what you are thankful for (one does the even numbers, the other the odd). Do this fun activity while taking a walk, a jog, riding in the car, or even while doing the dishes.
8. General thankfulness can be interspersed with health and fitness-related items, using the odd/even approach in step 7.

The law of attraction says that the more we appreciate, the more we will find *and have* to appreciate.

Meditation
Meditation is the act of stopping all conscious thought for a period of time. When we do this we discontinue all the disempowering contemplations that disconnect us from our True Self, Higher Self, Life Force, God — however we wish to express it. Without this roof-brain chatter, we become one with our Source of Beingness, the point of stillness from which all springs. Although we also stop all "positive" thoughts, the release from our destructive, mental ramblings allows us to connect with our Creator. During these few minutes, Life Force or Universal Intelligence is allowed to flow more fully to and through us, revitalizing us. In the process we also get out of the way so that our body/mind can heal itself without the detrimental effects of our resistance-producing, erroneous opinions and beliefs. In actuality, holding pure, positive thoughts for a few minutes would be just as effective as eliminating all conscious thoughts (meditation). However, for most of us it is far easier to hold no thoughts than it is to keep out all negative thoughts for even 30 seconds. For these

reasons, meditation (i.e., listening to or connecting with God/Universal Intelligence) is an effective tool for promoting our well-being. To meditate:

1. Find a quiet place.
2. Get comfortable and close the eyes or stare at an object, such as a lighted candle, to prevent thought-provoking visual stimulation. Sitting is better than lying so one doesn't fall asleep. Sleeping is not meditating.
3. Choose a word or two or a phrase to repeat during the length of the meditation, or just focus on your breathing. The words can be anything from religious to meaningless syllables. Silently say one word or phrase on inhalation and the same or a different word/phrase on the exhalation.
4. When your mind wanders, as it will for beginners, just bring it back gently (Don't beat up on yourself for straying).
5. Start with five minutes and gradually work up to fifteen or twenty minutes. Use a timer that dings or taps you on the shoulder when the time is up so you don't have to wonder or keep checking. At first, five minutes will seem like a lifetime or longer.
6. Stick with it. It is worth it and it does get easier and more enjoyable with practice. Studies have shown longtime meditators to be much healthier, as a group, than the general population. They experience significant decreases in pain, depression, anxiety, blood pressure and other maladies; thus meditators require less medication and fewer visits to the doctor.

Replace Bad Habits With Better Ones

Giving something up leaves a void in our life. If we don't replace a "bad" habit with another, more beneficial one, then we will probably eventually revert to our old ways and the joy *and problems it brought us.*

We can learn from Jerry Dunn, who gradually replaced his drug and alcohol habit with running, to become America's

105

Ed Mayhew with Mary Mayhew

Marathon Man and run 200 marathons in 2000. Or we can look to Dick Collins who was a 5'10", 240 pound, 2-pack-a-day smoker at age 42 when his doctor warned him of impending serious health risks. As a result, Dick replaced his bad-health habits with walking and running and went on to become a living legend in ultra-marathon racing, having at one time in his early fifties finished a string of 110 marathons and 77 ultras without a single DNF (Did Not Finish).

Before we give up a "vice" that has served us well (even though it has harmed us also) we must decide what we are going to substitute in its place. Where else can we find the joy that the "bad" habit obviously gave us? Maybe we can take up: gardening, rock climbing, woodworking, whittling, playing a musical instrument, cooking more nutritious foods, etc.

Relax And Enjoy Life

Stress is good. It helps us meet our deadlines, complete important projects, and pass tests of one kind or another.

It also prepares us to successfully fight or run away when danger presents itself. The body marshalls all its resources so it can take the physical action needed for survival. It has been programmed into us since the day of the saber-tooth tiger.

However, now we live in a different world — a relatively sedentary one due to the much-appreciated convenience of fax machines, heating thermostats, computers and remote controls. We seldom need to do battle with tigers and other beasts anymore save for an occasional pesky fly or mosquito. The dangers we perceive now deal with bumper-to-bumper traffic, hectic lifestyles, business deadlines, and people in our personal space with whom we don't always see eye to eye. In these situations it is not usually appropriate to physically fight or run away when we get stressed, especially if we want to keep our job, live with our family, and stay off the evening news. Without the physical outlets of the evolutionary past, our stresses can go on hour after hour, day after day. When these stresses linger for long periods of time, they can easily become detrimental to our health and general well being. The bodily resources that would be used for digesting food; battling viruses, bacteria, and cancer cells; and repairing and renewing cells are tied up in preparedness to do battle with an enemy that cannot be fought.

106

Stress is a *perception*, not an event. My daughters and I love to ride roller coasters; my wife won't go near one. Why? When my wife thinks about coasters, she focuses on the dangers and potential discomforts. The rest of the family thinks about how much fun and how exciting the ride will be.

One person sees a situation at work as a problem, a headache; another sees it as an exhilarating *challenge*. Passenger B whiteknuckles her flight across the country, while passenger D enjoys the convenience and amenities of air travel.

The key and most important element is always the focus. What we focus upon makes all the difference. Two men in prison cells side by side look out through their bars. One focuses on the mud on the grounds and feels the despair of his situation. The other prisoner looks up at the stars and is filled with awe as he contemplates the size, grandeur, majesty, and meaning of the heavens.

Relax and enjoy life. Frequently take time to notice what you are thinking about or focusing upon and how you are feeling. If what you are "looking at" is stressing you out, then choose a little better thought on the subject at hand or contemplate something *completely different*. If a problem has your attention, make sure you are focusing on solutions and not just rehashing over and over again the possible, dire consequences of the problem.

In her seventies Helen Klein can compete in 50 and 100-mile foot races because she focuses on her body and how it feels, not the obstacles or difficulty of the race. Helen notices if her body is tensing or tightening up and if her bio-mechanics are faltering in order to concentrate on keeping her muscles relaxed and agile so as to stay the course to the distant finish line. Our 87-year-old amateur contortionist, June Tatro, uses muscle tensing/relaxing techniques and deep breathing exercises to stay supple and instructs her 80, 90, and 95-year-old students in her fitness classes in the same. If Helen and June have used muscle-relaxation techniques (including yoga for Helen) to become Masters of *FA50*, then maybe we can no doubt benefit from them, too. Here are seven ways to relax your body for a fitter you:

1. Breathing — A prerequisite for Being Fitter After 50

Think of something that makes you angry. Maybe it's a driver just sitting there when the light turns green or perhaps that person in the express lane at the supermarket searching for her checkbook *after* her 21 products (with a 15-item limit clearly posted) have been rung up. Whatever it is, *feel* the anger it generates in you! Pretend that this anger-producing scenario is playing out right now. Take about 30 seconds to experience this event in your imagination. Notice what your breathing is like when you are feeling this hostility.

Now switch gears and get in touch with something that makes you sad or depressed. Maybe it's seeing a child who has a terminal disease. Whatever it is, take half a minute to *feel* the sadness and notice what this does to your breathing. Was your breathing the same as it was when you were angry?

Think about something exciting. Focus on a person or event that makes you happy, thrilled, passionate. Notice the inhalations and exhalations now.

Finally, remember what it is like to lie in a hammock in the shade with a gentle summer breeze caressing you, or what a good massage feels like. As you relax into the hammock or melt into the magic fingers, pay attention to your breathing.

Did your breathing pattern change for each of these scenarios you just played out? You bet it did. Different types of breathing and our emotions are intricately weaved together. When our mood changes, so does our breathing. One cannot stay angry while enjoying relaxed, deep breathing. Thus is the power of learning deep-breathing techniques. Performers use deep breathing before going on stage; athletes take a breath before shooting free throws or starting their high jump approach. It's that powerful.

Remember, negative emotions pinch off the Life Force that created our bodies and sustains them. In our often-hectic, fast-paced lives, we tend to breath shallowly and in our upper chest area. This type of tense breathing limits the amount of life-giving oxygen being delivered to the cells of our body and causes a level of stress that interferes with the repair and renewal of the trillions upon trillions of cells of which we are made. By consciously practicing deep breathing while driving, sitting in meetings, waiting in lines, and getting ready for work, we can eliminate some of the excess stress that is preventing us from being fitter after 50. We get some of the invigorating, deep breathing during aerobic workouts, but we can't just get up in the middle of an important and stress-producing meeting and go for a run; we *can* do deep breathing inconspicuously from time to time during the meeting.

Begin by lying on your back on a bed or soft carpet (no, not during the business meeting). Place a book on your stomach (*Gone With The Wind* would be good, but any book with a good plot and interesting characters will do). Exhale as much air from your lungs as possible by squeezing your stomach toward your spine. Notice the book sinking down with your belly. Now breathe in trying to fill your abdominal area first and see how high you can raise the book (no hands, please). Once the stomach area is expanded fully, you can attempt to fill the chest. Do this several times, focusing on the raising and lowering of the book. Once you have this pattern down you can practice while seated (without the book). Breathe in fairly vigorously through the nose and then relax as you exhale through pursed lips and finally tighten the abdomen to force the last bit of air out. Do this refreshing, stress-relieving technique several times a day for at least 30 days — until it becomes a habit, but don't stress over it. It should be enjoyable and relaxing, not another stressor in your life.

2. The Progressive Relaxation Technique

Lie comfortably on your bed or in a recliner. Tense the muscles in your left leg and foot while breathing in deeply. When you have a full inhalation, hold your breath for a second and then silently tell your left leg and foot to relax optimally while you exhale gently. Focus on your left leg as you relax it and feel the warmth in it. Next, repeat the above for the right leg and foot. Continue this process for the hip area; the thoracic area (chest, back and stomach); left arm and hand; right arm and hand; shoulders; and finally, the head, neck and face. Then take a deep breath while tightening the muscles of the whole body, followed by exhaling gently while relaxing the muscles starting at the head and slowly allowing the wave of relaxation to flow all the way down to the feet. Do this full-body relaxation two more times. Now continue breathing deeply while staying relaxed from head to toe and thinking about something pleasant (e.g., skiing, soaking in a hot tub, floating on a beautiful lake, etc.) for five minutes or as long as you are enjoying your mini-vacation. Do this at least once a day until you can do this technique while sitting at your desk or in a waiting room (a non-conspicuous version). etc.

3. Get A Massage

The body's largest organ is the skin. A good massage increases the blood flow to this prominent organ, bringing vital nutrients and taking away toxins for healthy, radiant skin. An effective massage stimulates the body's own internal pharmacy to produce hormones, enzymes, and antibodies to promote our well-being. Of course, it also feels good and relaxes us.

4. Nothing Like A Good Soaking

Soaking in a hot tub or a bubble bath is an excellent way to relax and let the Life Force flow to and through us.

5. Making Love

After love making, the body relaxes and a sound, replenishing sleep often ensues. Loving, intimate relations is a superb stress releaser, among other things.

6. Aroma, Music and Color Therapy

Relaxation can be enhanced by the use of aroma therapy in the form of scented candles, bath oils, etc. In this vein, soothing music can set the mood for a good rest, as can color therapy, as in certain colored or muted lighting and full-spectrum lighting.

7. Catching a Wink or Two

The body is "torn down" during intense and long-duration exercise. It is only during the post-exercise rest cycle that the muscles and body in general are built stronger, more fit.

A major part of this recuperation phase is sleep. How much sleep one needs is an individual matter. A creative genius in the midst of a project, such as writing a book or sculpting a statue, can get by with two or three hours of sleep a night for relatively long periods of time, whereas a stressed-out person may need 10 or 11 hours a night or more. The best way to tell how much sleep you need is to notice how you feel with differing amounts under a variety of circumstances. Then, to be your best, abide by your particular "requirement," realizing that the amount needed will change from time to time.

Naps are an excellent tool for performing at our peak. Author and ultra runner John Medinger gives an example of Dick Collins' (see chapter 2) famous 10-minute naps. One year

Dick and John were running the Angeles Crest 100-Miler when at about 4 A.M. Dick said he was really tired and needed a nap. So they found a soft spot next to the trail and as soon as Dick lay down, before John could even say "nighty-night; don't let the bedbugs bite," he was sound asleep. After about 10 minutes, refreshed, they resumed their run. The nap must have done the job, because Dick finished strong for his best ever time at Angeles Crest.

It is important to state your intent for the benefit of your biological alarm clock, before you lie down; that is, to affirm that this is just going to be a nap, not sleep, and that it will be so many minutes long or to a certain time. Otherwise you can wake up groggy and worse off than before you lay down because the mind/body thought it was the beginning of sleep time and the short "sleep" is a rude awakening; or you can accidently sleep through an important deadline. It is critical that you also program your mind that your intention and belief is that the 10-minute, 20-minute, or ... *nap* will be invigorating and rejuvenating.

Whistle While You Work

Besides being relaxing, music can stimulate us to take action. Have a ready stash of songs/music (CD's and tapes) that get your adrenaline flowing. Not only can you use this music during your workouts to maximize your effort, but equally significant is the playing of the music before a workout (or other activity for which you need to be energized) to get you "out the door." When we are worn out from the mental stresses of the day, this stimulating music can mean the difference between deciding, "I'm too exhausted to exercise today — I need my rest more;" and "yes, I want to do this — I can do this!" Keep in mind that with today's lifestyles we are seldom *physically* tired from our busy schedule. We are usually mentally and emotionally stressed/worn out and vigorous, physical movement is the best thing for this. If individuals over the age of 50, such as Helen Klein and Dick Collins can compete in 24-hour races and 6-day racing events, and others, such as Denver Fox, are taking 100 and 200-mile biking excursions in the Rocky Mountains, then my body can take a 30-minute workout TODAY!

Picture This

Don't underestimate the power of a picture. We know what they say: "A picture is worth a thousand push-ups." (or something like that)

When comedian Jerry Lewis was preparing for his Broadway stage debut in *Damn Yankees*, around age 70, he was grossly overweight. He knew he couldn't stand up to the rigors of daily live performances unless he lost weight. He got a picture of himself when he was younger and the exact weight he now desired to be again. He taped this picture of himself at his "ideal" weight to his treadmill machine. Each morning he would spend an hour or so on the treadmill while staring at this svelte, younger Lewis. The day the show opened he weighed exactly the same as he had when the picture was taken — his goal.

Post pictures where you'll see them of the way you want to look, what you want to do, or of people who have the energy you desire. Paste a picture of your head/face on a picture of the body of your dreams which you can find in a magazine, a photo album, etc. Find a picture of yourself when you looked the way you would like to look now or had the fitness level you would like to regain. Stick up pictures of places you will travel to and things you will do when you are fitter. Put these pictures where you will see them during your everyday activities, your workouts, and even when you get up in the morning and hit the sack at night.

Take "before" pictures in skimpy attire that will gross you out and heighten your desire to take significant action. Take follow-up pictures every month or two to show your progress and motivate you to stick with your new lifestyle. Adjust your program and make changes if the pictures don't show sufficient improvement.

Partner Up

Some of us can go it alone. Others need companions on their journey to a fiiter self. Recruit a workout partner. It may mean the difference between your sticking with your new exercise/eating program and quitting. Not wanting to let your friend down by cancelling your joint workout can be just the incentive you need to hang in there until your new program becomes a firmly-established habit. The support and encouragement you give each other may make all the difference and develop or strengthen a lifelong friendship.

Ruth Anderson and Dick Collins worked out and traveled to competitions together. Terry Hitchcock recruited his family to help him in his 2,000-mile run from Minneapolis to Atlanta to help motherless children. Paul Reese had his wife's support, assistance, and company on his coast-to-coast trek across the U.S., and then across each state in the union. James Hill does his speed work with a running club. Our master bikers joined biking clubs for support and technical expertise and our swimmers linked up with swim teams for the same reasons.

Get a Personal Trainer

If you have very little experience with working up a sweat or lifting weights, then finding a certified personal trainer who specializes in helping people in your age group is one of the best things you could do. If finances are an issue, then you can get a trainer for just the first few months or for only one workout every two weeks. Another option is to have a trainer for just your strength sessions and do your aerobic workouts on your own.

A good trainer will get you started right, keep you safe, motivate you for optimal results and make sure you do each exercise correctly for maximum return on your effort. Or you could just talk with knowledgeable, enthusiastic exercisers (preferably those close to your age) who can give you free guidance and would be eager to do so. They are just waiting for you to ask.

Races And Special Events

Most of our friends and trailblazers in chapters 2 and 3 used races as their motivation to get fitter after 50. Remember, 54-year-old Helen Klein had never raced nor had any interest in foot races until she finally experienced the thrill of racing. Lois Lindsay, at 42, had never biked. Yet, once she was hit by the racing bug she went on to become a National Cycling Champion in her fifties. The last thing on Sister Madonna Buder's mind in her late forties would have been competing in triathlons. But once she started competing, she likewise caught the fever, and by age 70 had raced in over 200 triathlons — not bad for a non-athletic nun. The moral of these vignettes is that we should not dismiss racing as inspiration to get into shape no matter how old we are or how little interest we *think* we have.

Besides racing there are special events that can be your reason to work out and eat well. A backpacking trip on the Appalachian Trail (like my wife and I took years ago) and bike tours to see and experience the countryside firsthand are other options. How about getting fit enough to ride the whitewater of the mighty Colorado River or hike the majestic Swiss Alps, like Janet Baker-Murray did recently. There is no end to the events we can get in shape to enjoy. Of course, there are the old standbys, wedding days, class reunions, and summer trips to the beach.

Decide on a challenge commensurate with your current fitness level. Pick something you really believe, with some training, you can achieve; but at the same time, make sure it is challenging enough to inspire you. Talk to someone *who is fit* and around your age to get an idea of what you may be capable.

Once you've chosen an appropriate goal, commit to it by paying the entry fee right away, purchasing the airline tickets (if needed) and telling those around you what you are going to do. Also, you can write up a contract or agreement with yourself as to what you are planning. Maybe a friendly wager with your mate, brother or friend will keep you from quitting when obstacles arise, as they surely will. Would combining your challenge with raising money for a favorite charity help keep you motivated. Might you, for instance, participate in a walk-a-thon or run a marathon as a member of Team Diabetes or ...

A Contract With Myself

Make a written commitment to yourself. Decide exactly what you are going to do. For example, you might commit to run 3 days per week, eat 5 fruits and vegetables a day, make a list of 100 things you appreciate each Sunday night, or ... Write down your decision, sign it, date it, and have a witness sign it, too. Then post it where you will see it regularly. There is something magical about having made a written commitment to — a contract with — one's self. Our word, our trustworthiness is on the line. We have a "legal" binding contract with ourself and breaking it has serious consequences. Doesn't it?

Affirmations

An affirmation is a statement, a positive assertion, that is repeated over and over. Helen Klein uses affirmations to keep her body relaxed and her biomechanics correct in order to complete ultra-long runs, such as 50 and 100-mile races.

An example of an affirmation could be, "I am healthy!" However, if we don't believe that because we are actually sick and know it, then it is not going to help us. For an affirmation to be successful, it is essential that it be said with strong positive emotions. We must believe it. A better affirmation, one that we might believe, could be, "My body has the ability to heal itself. I am allowing it to do so!" If we can believe this statement, then repeating it with strong, positive feelings while relaxing or doing aerobic exercise can be beneficial. At the very least, by focusing on this statement, negative, deleterious thoughts about our well-being are kept at bay for the duration of the affirming. In the best case scenario, your excitement, a positive emotion concerning this truth, can open the way for the Life Force that created and maintains the body to flow more fully to and through the cells of the body and bring it back into balance (i.e., ease versus dis-ease).

Some sample affirmations are:

"land lightly," "relax and move," or "shoulders back and down" — Helen Klein's directives to herself as she runs

"I am getting stronger!"

"Relax, all is well."

"Thank you mind, and body, for everything."

"I appreciate my trillions of cells, which know what to do and do it well."

Try this affirmation technique when you wake up in the morning, while driving, or during walks/runs: Think of a time when you felt absolutely great. For me, such a time was playing tag on ice skates as a teen at the local *Rocky Woods* frozen pond. Use this wonderful feeling/event of *yours* each time you do this powerful affirmation. With a big smile plastered on your face, silently say, "Relax and" while exhaling; then, "let it in" while inhaling; next, "the Rocky Woods" on the exhalation; and finally, "feeling" on the inhalation. Repeat this affirmation for several minutes while conjuring up and re-experiencing as much of the positive feeling as you can. Be ever mindful that it is not the words themselves, but the *feeling* that they illicit, in regards to the subject you've chosen or your general well-being, that manifests results.

Take In A Movie

Have a small library of movies that you can plunk into the DVD or VCR that will ignite your burning desire to be fit. This is not meant to be a regular occurrence. This set of videos/DVDs is for when the impetus to take care of yourself has been lost; when you no longer find it easy to get up and do your workouts. This is when a *Rocky (I, II, III, IV,or V), Chariots of Fire, Body for Life* (see chapter 8), *October Sky, Space Cowboys, Crouching Tiger - Hidden Dragon*, etc. movie can get you up off the couch, out the door and excited about your workouts and where they are taking you.

Savings Bonds - The Motivator

Tell your son or daughter that you are going to give your grandchild (their son or daughter) a $50 or $100 U.S. Saving's Bond each of the next 3 to 6 months *if* you stick with a new exercise program or train for and run in an upcoming race. If the child is old enough, you can let him know, too, that you are giving the bonds for his college education, ... This process puts the pressure on yourself to carry through with your goal until the exercise habit is well-established. Bonds are good because they cost only half of their face value. This makes them a more impressive gift, that is very affordable and encourages saving in order to get the full value.

Diet For A More Charitable America

Make a commitment to give a dollar or ... to your favorite charity for each serving of fruits, vegetables and whole grains you eat over a given period of time. For instance, ten servings a day for thirty days would raise $300 for a worthy cause while motivating you to eat more healthfully. Put a limit on how much you will give so you can be comfortable with the challenge. This is a win-win situation. If you are worried that all this food will "blimpasize" you, remember that Helen Klein maintains her weight around 109 pounds while eating 10 to 12 servings of f & v a day.

The Wheel of Fitness

Focusing on what we want and why we want it is the secret to lifelong fitness.Here is a technique that flat-out works!

Draw a two or three-inch diameter circle in the middle of a blank eight-and-a-half-by-eleven piece of paper. In the middle of the circle put the words, "Fitter After 50." Now traveling around the outside of the circle, like the numbers on a clock, write the reasons why you wish to be *FA50*. Starting at the 1:00 o'clock position, write the first reason that comes to mind and then draw a line from the reason to the *FA50* circle. Move to the 2:00 position and add a second reason, again with a line to the circle. Continue around the circle or "clock" until you have 12 reasons and lines. Now read the reasons out loud while putting an arrow point on the end of each line pointing toward the circle. Starting at 1:00, read them in this fashion: "I choose to be fitter after 50 because I don't want to be a burden on my children and grandchildren." Then you might say, "I choose to be FA50 because I desire to have the energy and stamina to travel the U.S. and the world." After you've gone around the circle stating all your 12 reasons, say, "That is why I am going to enjoy being fitter after 50!" Relax and enjoy this exercise. The object is to focus our attention on the reasons why we want to be FA50 so as to strengthen our resolve and belief that we can and will. Make sure that the great majority of the reasons address what you want — not what you don't want.

This activity is based on a technique presented in the works of Abraham-Hicks. Go to www.abraham-hicks.com for other techniques and the Art of Allowing.

CHAPTER 5 RESEARCHERS STUMBLE UPON THE FOUNTAIN OF YOUTH

Man has searched for the Fountain of Youth since time immemorial. Finally, modern researchers have located it. As one would suspect, it was right under our noses all the time. This magic bullet is impressive, to say the least. It has been shown in scientific studies (clinical, double blind, longitudinal, etc) to:

- delay and prevent diabetes, colon cancer, heart disease, stroke, and osteoporosis
- improve and increase stamina, agility, strength, power, flexibility, and endurance
- improve balance and lessen the number of falls
- increase the peak oxygen capacity or volume of the lungs (VO2)
- increase lean body mass while decreasing body fat
- speed up the metabolism and increase the number of calories burned while at rest (even while sleeping)
- prevent or lessen the severity of migraine headaches
- decrease stress and prevent stress-related ailments (lessens the production of the stress hormone — cortisol)
- improve immune function by increasing the number and activity level of killer cells, T cells, white blood cells, ... thus protecting from infectious disease and foreign object invasion
- improve blood lipid profile
- control cholesterol by lowering dangerous LDL and increasing beneficial HDL
- lower resting heart rate
- stabilize blood sugar levels
- improve reaction time
- stimulate the sex drive
- make one feel and look younger
- boost self esteem and self confidence
- improve clarity of thinking
- stimulate the production of human growth hormone to levels more closely associated with youth

- **And scratch that itch where you can't reach it —
well, maybe that's a stretch**

What is this magic potion, and where can we get it? Or where is this miracle, mineral-water spring that we can soak in to be restored to our pimply days of yore?

It is neither an ancient, recently-discovered underground spring nor the latest multi-million-dollar miracle cure from our pharmacological labs nor even a witch doctor's mysterious brew from the rain forests of Peru. It's been right in front of us all these years, so close that we overlooked it. We were hoping for something more glamorous, something easy like a pill we could pop into our mouths like candy. What our scientists have uncovered (and continue to unearth, piece by piece) is plain old muscular movement, or what modern man calls "exercise."

Let me explain. We were designed by our Creator to need physical movement in order to function optimally, and through the eons movement and life itself have gone hand in hand. However, in recent years (especially the last 50 or so), the need and even the *inclination* to self-propel ourselves with old fashioned, muscular effort has been engineered out of our lives. As a result, chronic diseases, such as heart disease, cancer, osteoporosis, and diabetes are running rampant. Our ancestors did not live long lives despite getting plenty of exercise because there was limited medical knowledge, no cures for infectious diseases, and high mortality rates during childbirth and young childhood.

I remember rolling up windows on the car with a primitive hand crank, walking across the room to change channels, and getting up to answer the phone. Can you believe all the energy people had to expend just to survive way back in the pre-civilized world of the 1970's and 80's? Imagine living just 100 years ago when they had to chop and tote their firewood and constantly stoke the fire so it wouldn't go out; pump and carry their water by the bucketsful; and walk to school, work and town. Some of us complain when we have to get up to change the thermostat and absolutely panic, when we can't find the remote.

119

Is exercise really the fountain of youth that I have painted? Let's look at a few of the scientifiic studies and what some experts are saying.

Age specialist Walter M. Bortz, M.D., said it best when he wrote in the Journal of the American Medical Association, **"There is no drug in current or prospective use that holds as much promise for sustained health as a lifetime program of physical exercise. If you take a master sheet of paper and record on it all the changes in the human body that we ascribed to aging — changes in muscles, bones, brain, cholesterol, blood pressure, sleep habits, sexual performance, psychological inventory — and compile a similar list of changes due to physical inactivity, you will note a striking similarity between the 2 lists. The near duplication of the lists shows that many of the bodily changes we have always ascribed to the normal aging process are in fact caused by disuse."** Reprinted with permission from *It's Never Too Late!,* Breakaway Books (BreakAwayBooks.com).

Miriam E. Nelson, Ph.D., renowned researcher at the Tufts University Center on Aging has written regarding one of her peer-reviewed studies in the Journal of American Medical Association, "We found that after a year of strength training twice a week, older women's bodies were 15 to 20 years younger." Specifically, these women had regained muscle and bone while losing fat; they were re-energized and thus they became as active in their everyday lives as they had been years ago.

National columnist, Bard Lindeman, who writes "In Your Prime" for and about those of us 50 and older writes, "... (Exercise Is Your Ticket to the Longer Life Worth Living): Many of the effects of aging are, in fact, the end products of disuse ... The lesson in this essay is simply this — if you want to ensure a miserable old age, don't exercise."

Finally, Gary Hunter, Ph.D., professor of human studies and researcher at the University of Alabama exclaims, "Strength training is the closest thing to a fountain of youth."

Now you've heard what the experts are saying and I hear what you are saying, "Talk is cheap. Let's see some of the scientific findings that prove your point, Ed." Well, as luck would have it, I just happen to have some right here next to my computer. Fancy that!

As recently as the 1980s it was generally believed by the scientific community that losing muscle and strength was an irreversible component of aging. Then in the mid-eighties, groundbreaking research at the Tufts University Center On Aging shattered this mindset and showed that the loss of strength as we age is mainly the result of lifestyle choices — not a sign of aging. Scientists Walter Frontera, M.D., and William Evans, Ph.D., took 60 and 70-year-old men and put them through 12 weeks of high-intensity weight training at 80% of capacity on their lifts. Previous to this, researchers had checked out light lifting, that is, 50% and less of maximum, with middle-aged and older subjects and had only gotten poor results. By using greater resistance, more in line with what young adult males use to get stronger, they got excellent results, similar to what younger lifters get. The muscles of these 60 and 70-year-olds became 10 to 12 percent larger and 100 to 175 percent stronger. Most of these older men claimed that they were now *stronger than they had ever been.*

Maria Fiatarone, M.D., another staff member of the Tufts Center on Aging, decided that if high-intensity strength training worked with those in their sixties and seventies, then it should really help the frailest of the frail - 80 and 90-year-old nursing home residents. She rounded up six women and four men volunteers, ages 86 to 96. These were typical nursing home patients with at least two serious disease conditions each (including heart disease, diabetes, and osteoporosis). After lifting weights three times per week for 8 weeks, they had increased their strength by an average of 175 percent; their balance and walking speed improved by 48 percent.

Also from the Tufts Center, Miriam E. Nelson, Ph.D., and colleagues studied women ages fifty to seventy to see what effect strength training might have on bone density as it relates to protection from the ravages of osteoporosis. The study found that after one year of weight training the participants had gained one percent bone mass while a control group that didn't exercise lost a whopping two percent of their bone density. But that's not all! The strength-trained women also had:

1. Fourteen percent improvement in their balance ability scores
2. Become 27 percent more active (more recreational activities, stair climbing, ...)
3. Lost inches and dropped dress sizes
4. Improved flexibilty

In yet more studies at the Tufts Center on Aging (they sure are a busy bunch), strength training was found to help those with moderate-to-severe rheumatoid arthritis by decreasing pain, restoring strength and muscle, and improving range of motion. Patients with osteoporosis of the knee, after four months of at-home strength training, had forty percent improvement in joint function, a fifty percent increase in strength, and reported forty-three percent less pain.

Just to show that Tufts is not the only research center to find strength training of great benefit for the mature, here are the results of a six-month study at the University of Alabama. These strength-trained 61 to 77-year-olds gained 4.5 pounds of lean tissue while losing 6 pounds of fat. This revved up their metabolism causing them to burn, on average, 230 more calories per day — even on days they didn't exercise.

A study of 707 non-smoking men reported in the New England Journal of Medicine found that those who walked more than 2 hours per day had, compared to their peers, half the risk of dying. Scientists conducting this study at Wageningen University in the Netherlands came to the conclusion that exercise boosts the immune system in the elderly helping them fight off infections. The study looked at the effect of exercise and/or vitamin-enriched foods on the immune system of 112 men and women. While exercise was shown to be significant in helping the frail and inactive elderly to fight infectious disease, the vitamin-enriched products had little effect.

We all know we should exercise on a regular basis, but many of us just don't for one reason or another. In chapter 1 we were reminded of how we will benefit from working out and we just read some of the scientific bases. Let's see if we can blast some of our excuses out of the water and strengthen our resolve that we can and will take *good* care of ourselves. Here are some excuses you may recognize.

Too Busy — More Important Things To Do

It takes time to deal with a debilitating, chronic disease or condition that is sucking the life out of us (and the joy out of life) because we were too busy through the years to take care of ourselves — to exercise. Are we really too busy to get the physical movement our body craves? Dick Collins (chapter 2) could have made the excuse that he was too busy, and actually, he did for many years before he took up running to improve his health. Dick ran his own contracting firm while helping his wife, Barbara, raise five children. Yet, he found time to run 40 to 50 miles during the week as training and 1,037 races (mostly during the weekends) including 238 ultras and 163 marathons over a 21-year period. On top of this overflowing schedule, when he wasn't actually running *in* the races he was *running* the races (either as an official or assisting the runners or helping out in any way he could). According to his friend Tim Skopphammer, "People from all over called him [Dick] wanting to know about courses and how to train. He'd always take the time to talk, call them back or write them."

But we don't need to run 6-day races, marathons, or even 5K races like Dick did to get and stay in shape. Dr. Glenn A. Gaesser at the University of Virginia has shown that just two or three easily managed 10-minute exercise breaks per day is all we need. In 2000, Dr. Gaesser studied 40 mostly-middle-aged adults exercising a mere 10 minutes at a time, only 15 times per week. The exercise consisted of things such as taking short walks, dancing around one's home, lifting dumb bells at the office, and stretching. Here's what he found on average after a scant three weeks:

- Aerobic capacity improved 10 to 15 percent — to a level equivalent to that of a typical individual 10 to 15 years younger
- Strength and muscular endurance improved 40 to 100 percent, or to the level of a person 20-years younger
- Flexibility scores improved to that of individuals 20 years younger
- An average of 3 pounds were lost — a healthy rate of loss of one pound per week

• Cholesterol and triglyceride levels dropped significantly

You can read more about what Dr. Gaesser calls The Sparks Program in chapter 8 — Eight That Work. The above shows that we can fit exercise into our schedule no matter how jam-packed our life is by breaking our workouts into bite-size chunks that we won't choke on. In the end, fitting life-giving movement into our lives is a matter of making it a priority. And if we can't seem to quite make our health a priority, then we probably need to reevaluate our life. After all, if we lose our health then all the other "more important" stuff will take a backseat, anyway.

Don't Know How To Start

Go to your front door and turn the little knob, open the door and step outside and just keep stepping (also called taking a walk). If you have been very sedentary, five minutes may do. Now that wasn't so bad, was it? So you *do* know how to get started, after all.

James Hill, at 54, didn't know what to do either when he had high blood pressure and a sedentary lifestyle, but decided to give running a shot. His procedure was to read some books on the subject and later join a running club where he found some runners he could run with and learn from once a week. But first he just started running in his neighborhood. Seven or so years later, he's one of the top American marathoners in his age group. Lois Lindsay didn't know how to ride a bike when she decided in her forties to take up cycling. She borrowed a bike and taught herself how to ride it. Then she got advice from her son and husband (avid bikers both) and joined a cycling club for more assistance. Now in her sixties, she's a cycling champion.

In chapters 8 and 10 I give you fitness programs that work and will get you started off right, and sources of information on how to get started (mostly web sites). Or you can visit your local video store and rent or buy an exercise video/DVD and get started right away. Even easier and perhaps quicker, would be to check your TV listings for exercise shows and learn from the TV fitness experts while you follow along. And there's always your local library or book store. It is really not hard to start once you make the decision to do it.

Might Get Hurt Or Worse

You might get hurt, sick, or worse if you don't get moving. In truth, we are more likely to run into health problems if we don't get up off the couch and spend some time with a dumbbell (and I'm not talking about your husband, ladies).

We've seen that the researchers at leading universities are studying the effects of intense weight training on frail 80 and 90-year-old nursing home residents; a significant fact here is that they are not reporting any *cardiovascular events or injuries.* The American College of Sports Medicine now recommends strength training for *all* individuals over 50. Of course, getting medical clearance from your doctor or other health professional if there is *any* reason for you to wonder about your ability to withstand an exercise program is the smart thing to do. Also, finding a certified and personable personal trainer with experience with "older" exercisers, is a wise way to get you started off on the right foot. Getting instructions from an expert in how to best exercise aerobically and how to use strength-training machines and weights correctly is an excellent way to prevent needless injuries and get the most out of your time in the gym. There are aquatic exercise classes and Tai Chi for lessening the stress and strain on arthritic joints and the like.

If there were a group that we would think needed to avoid vigorous exercise, it would probably be those with chronic obstructive pulmonary disease (COPD — e.g., asthma, emphysema, ...). Yet in a peer- reviewed study (Archives of Physical Medicine and Rehabilitation. January 2000;81:102-9) by M. Gimenez and colleagues it was found that COPD patients did better with maximally-tolerated 45-minute aerobic training than a similar group did with moderate exercise. Patients in the high-intensity aerobics group significantly reduced dyspnea (difficult or labored breathing) at rest while increasing peak oxygen consumption (VO2) and work capacity. No adverse health events occurred during the training program for either of the two groups.

This is not to encourage those with emphysema and other COPD's to go out and try to run a mile. This program was under strict medical supervision. It does point out that under proper conditions (sometimes medically supervised) and with the appropriate level of exercise, just about anyone, no matter what his handicap or condition, can get in health-enhancing workouts. Remember, Terry Hitchcock had a heart attack while training for his 2,000-mile trek for the children and then received clearance from his doctors to take his ultra, ultra run and completed it successfully. By starting slowly at a level of exercise commensurate with our fitness status, listening to our body, and getting the advice of fitness and/or medical experts, we can exercise safely at any age, no matter what our condition.

I'm Too Old

Our friends from chapters 2 and 3 would like a word with us. Norm Green, our Pennsylvania minister, would like to remind us that he ran a 2-hour and 27-minute and 42-second marathon at age 55; that's well under 6 minutes per mile. Most 20-year-olds could not keep pace for even a quarter of a mile! The marathon overall world record is 2 hours and 5 minutes and change. Warren Utes wants to add his 3:18:10 marathon at age 75 to the mix. That means Warren ran about 7 minutes and 45 second miles for 26 miles. Wow! It's safe to say that more than 95 percent of American 20-year-olds could not run 7:45 for a single, solitary mile. As for the ladies, let me add that in the 50 to 54 age bracket, Ruth Anderson ran a 50-mile race in 7 hours, 10 minutes, and 58 seconds. My mathematical computations figure that to be just over 8:40/mile for 50 miles. Not to be outdone, Helen Klein clocks in with a 9:01:38 for the 50-miler at age 60-plus (under 11 minutes a mile) and 4:31 for a marathon at age 75. But they are just kids, interjects Peter Jurczyk; at 91, I was doing mile swims during my 3 or 4-times-per-week training sessions.

Although these master champions of fitness didn't actually ask me to relay the above accomplishments, I'm sure if they were here, Norm, Warren, Ruth, Helen, and Peter would all want you to know and come to the conclusion that you are never too old to benefit from exercise.

Turning our attention to strength training, the American Heart Association Science Advisory Committee on February 22, 2000 published their review of the effects of resistance training. Their conclusion was that moderate to high intensity strength training two to three times per week for three to six months increases strength and endurance by 35 to 100 percent in men and women of *all ages.*

Let's face it, we all age, but we don't have to become decrepit and fall apart. Science has shown that lifestyle changes, such as appropriate exercise, can increase our body's production of human growth hormone, reversing its usual decline as we age; and maintaining high levels of HGH is at the center staying "youthful." Frailty and feebleness in old age is not a natural part of aging — it may be common or even seem normal, but it is not necessary. If it were, then 75-year-old grandmothers such as Helen Klein wouldn't run in and complete 100-mile mountain trail races. No sirree Bob!

Won't Make Any Real Difference

At age 55, Robert Beal, a rotund, 245-pound, 2-pack-a-day smoker, decided to give cycling a go. Seventeen years later, he was a trim ex-smoker who would regularly ride his bike 300 miles a week and was employed by the United States Cycling Federation as a trainer of up-and-coming U.S. cycling stars. Ask Robert if exercise made a difference in his life!

In strength training studies there were frail 80 and 90-year-olds who reclaimed enough of their leg strength to be able to throw away their canes and/or walkers Ask them if weight training made a difference in their lives!

My own 90-year-old mother was having trouble getting out of her chair, a condition that was threatening her ability to live independently in her own apartment. She would struggle to get up, needing several efforts to finally stand. With just a couple of minutes of leg exercises 3 times a week and three 5-minute walks around her apartment, in just a few weeks she was able to get out of her chair in a single bound. Well, maybe "bound" is the wrong word, but you get the picture. The bottom line is, she can control her own destiny and stay in her home, perhaps for years to come. Ask my mother if this little bit of exercise made a difference!

I have always enjoyed the challenge of seeing how many chin-ups I could do (you know, where you jump up and grab a horizontal bar or tree limb and see how many times you can pull your chin up over the bar). In my early thirties I set a record of 30 in a row. At age 54, with just over two hours of strength training per week, I was able to beat my best ever by 33% with a new personal best of 40. That may not be as important as being able to walk independently, getting out of a chair unaided, or training future Olympians, but it gave me great satisfaction and did make all the difference — to me!

Don't Like To Sweat

In the previous chapters we have met some regular folks who have accomplished remarkable feats of fitness. We have showcased them to remind us that we can get fitter with age, and that it's not a requirement of aging that we fall apart; *that* is completely optional. Nor do we have to compete with our Masters of Fitness to get fit ourselves; we don't have to kayak the length of the Mississippi, skip around the rim of the Grand Canyon, or mimic those professional basketball players sporting rivulets of sweat all over their bodies to improve our fitness. Most fitness experts will tell us that moderate exercise is sufficient to improve fitness. For example, Jo Ann Manson, Harvard Medical School, said something to the effect that the Nurses' Health Study found that women who regularly engaged in brisk walking decreased their risk of heart disease to the same degree as women who engaged in more vigorous exercise. One doesn't need to run a marathon.

We can bypass the sweating and heavy panting (save for any hanky panky on the side) by taking early morning walks in the summer, before the sun gets to its zenith, or strolling in an air-conditioned mall. Another option is swimming and aquatic aerobics.

The skin is our body's largest organ, and when we sweat, we are cleaning, cooling and eliminating titanic quantities of toxins and waste products from our bodies. In addition, a team of researchers at the University of Tubingen in Germany has recently discovered that when we sweat, the skin releases an antimicrobial chemical called dermcidin. This antibiotic protein was tested on four common species of bacterium and killed all four, including the potentially-lethal Escherichia coli and Staphylococcus aureus. It feels good to sweat when we get used to it and dress in appropriate workout clothes. Besides, if you are a woman you don't sweat, you just "glow," and men — well, we know about men.

Fear of Building Behemoth Muscles

Women don't have enough testosterone (a key hormone necessary for pronounced muscles) to build big, bulky muscles. Those women bodybuilders we see have not gotten that big (does the word grotesque come to mind) by just lifting a few weights. It might be safe to say that they are pharmacologically enhanced. Big, non-feminine muscles are definitely not something a woman thinking about strength training needs to be concerned about.

Men, if you are afraid of becoming "muscle bound" and having all that muscle interfere with your golf swing, then you have too much free time on your hands. You would have to get pretty fit and nice and muscular first. Once there, you can always stop at this nice and muscular plateau. The number of men who have a difficult time combing their hair because of protruding and overlapping muscle tissue is miniscule; especially in comparison with the number of protruding-and-overlapping-their-belt men. Or maybe you are afraid that after you've built all this muscle mass, you would get tired of training and stop, and all your muscle would turn into fat. Truth be known, it probably already has. Obviously, these worries are not a problem — just lame excuses.

I'm Fine (Happy) The Way I Am

Really? Have a friend or your mate take a picture of you in a standing, relaxed pose wearing the skimpiest of bathing suits. Then take a good look at the pictures. If you like them AND wouldn't mind posting them on your web page or putting them in the local newspaper, then maybe you are truly happy with the way you look. On the other hand, if the mere thought of letting anyone take a picture of you in a bikini, etc. is scary, then ...

Or just stand in front of a full-length mirror *au natural* (in a relaxed pose) and make an evaluation. That should tell you whether you are *really* fine with the way you look and the state of your body.

Maybe that all sounds too vain for a middle-ager, so let's turn our attention to energy levels. Do you have the energy that you had 10 years ago, or even just 5 years ago? Do you look forward to going out at night or flopping down on the sofa or your recliner? How are you at carrying a load up a couple of flights, or do you consider yourself load enough? Could you keep up with a six or seven-year-old at Disney World? How about keeping up with a grandchild or great-grandchild 10 or 20 years from now? Will you have the energy to enjoy them fully?

Do you have an ailment or two that you could do without? How are the numbers on your bloodwork? Triglycerides? Cholesterol? HDL's? LDL's? Blood pressure? Blood sugar? In most cases, any "numbers" that are causing you or your doctor concern can be normalized without supporting the pharmaceutical companies with your generous monthly "donations."

Too Much Trouble

If we really believed that just a couple of hours a week working out was going to make a jaw-dropping difference in our looks, make us feel like a kid again, and give us energy to enjoy our free time and do all the things we like, or used to like, to do — then we wouldn't think it was too much trouble. The real trouble is that our past half-hearted attempts at a make-over were such colossal busts that we no longer believe it can be done. What will reverse our defeatist attitude and revamp us from head to toe is doing the 60-Second Solution (chapter 7); choosing a program that works (chapter 8); and rereading the inspiring stories of our Masters of Fitness (chapters 2 & 3).

Exercise is only inconvenient and not worth the effort if it doesn't produce the goods; and this depends on our beliefs about exercise. Keep in mind that a belief is only a thought that one has thought so frequently or repeatedly that it has become a conviction. If the thoughts that birthed the belief were wrong, then the belief is ill-conceived and not serving us well. The 60-Second Solution is a potent tool for replacing our destructive, self-limiting thoughts and beliefs with empowering ones. Our fitness-pioneering friends in chapters 2 and 3 show us it can be done and that if they can do it, we can, too!

I'm Too Sick

I hear some of you: "I would BUT I have arthritis, asthma, heart disease, diverticulitis, osteoporosis, halitosis, toe fungus, and I weigh enough to pass for an elephant in the circus (which reminds me, I'm allergic to peanuts, too)." Those and others are not reasons not to exercise, but they are reasons *to* exercise. If we have a chronic, debilitating condition, we can use it as incentive, as impetus to begin a fitness program. Just make sure to get the okay and guidance of your health professional. The bottom line is that we can't afford not to exercise.

Let's look at the effects of a single workout. "Take a 50-year-old man who is somewhat overweight and typically has moderately elevated blood sugar, triglycerides, or blood pressure" says fitness expert William Haskell of the Stanford University Medical School. "A single bout of exercise of moderate intensity — like 30 to 40 minutes of brisk walking — will lower those numbers." And those improvements last for hours.

Now we turn our attention to some specific disease conditions and whether they make a good excuse (oops! I mean a good reason) to develop an intimate relationship with our sofa cushion.

1. * In a 1997 study at John Hopkins School of Medicine, six months of aerobic exercise on a treadmill increased the fitness of a group of 61 to 91-year-old heart patients by 22 percent. * The American Heart Association recommends strength training to lower one's heart rate and blood pressure. * According to a famous 1978 study of 20,000 Harvard University Alumni, middle-aged and older men who exercised moderately had just half the heart attacks of their sedentary contemporaries.
2. Asthmatics are helped by aerobic conditioning. Appropriate exercise increases lung capacity and strengthens the heart making it easier to take in oxygen and deliver it to the cells.
3. The Arthritis Foundation in its publications says that "exercise lessens pain, increases movement,

131

reduces fatigue and helps you look and feel better." Dynamic exercise, such as walking, cycling, and strength training, is good for those with arthritis. Dynamic exercise in one study was found to be superior to the usually recommended isometric and range-of-motion exercises; they improved muscle strength, physical conditioning, and joint mobility.

4. Appropriate, well-chosen abdominal and back exercises can reduce pressure on the lumbar discs in the lower back and increase circulation to get needed nutrients to the discs, thus reducing or eliminating lower back pain.

Whatever your excuse to take it easy, in actuality, it might be an even better reason why you would benefit from regularly-scheduled workouts.

Never Stick With It — Why Start?

That's a good question and I'm glad you are asking it. There are countless folks just like you and me who have yo-yo dieted, exercised on and off, and quit smoking numerous times over the years before they finally succeeded in:

A. Losing the weight *and keeping it off*
B. Getting in shape and staying in shape (i.e., sticking with a regular program of exercise)
C. Becoming a non-smoker for good

What made the difference is simply a decision, finally committing to a new and improved way of life. Usually, they got so low emotionally (so sick and tired of being sick and tired — so fed up with being fat — some would say they hit rock bottom) that they finally made that crucial commitment to change. Until then, their craving to eat junk food, crash on the couch, or blow smoke out of their noses was more attractive than their fledgling desire to change. The "bad" habit was too comfortable *and enjoyable*, even though they knew in their heart that it was bad for them and despite the fact that it also caused them considerable discomfort at other times.

The secret is to make it more compelling to go for a walk or run than to reach for yet another piece of chocolate cake.

We will share with you many ways to do this in chapter 7, The 60-Second Solution.

Until then, here are a couple of tricks you can use. First, what did Helen Klein do? She accepted a challenge that she wasn't originally very excited about, running a 10-mile race. What did most of our other Master mentors in chapters 2 and 3 do? They set themselves a challenge such as running or swimming in a race, going on a biking tour, or traveling a set distance to raise money for some worthy cause. They started small or relatively small (e.g., swimming the 50-meter backstroke, running in a 5K, etc.) and built up to longer, more arduous challenges. They *had* to train and get fitter and fitter in order to take on the ever-greater challenges. They didn't exercise to avoid heart disease, to lose 10 pounds, or get in shape (whatever that means). Those nebulous type of goals seldom work for long.

Find a race (biking, running, swimming, skating, ...); a walkathon to raise money for a charity; or a group bike tour (1,000 miles in 2 weeks, for instance) and commit to it. Sign up, pay the entry fee or down payment, write down your commitment, and tell everyone. Now you are "locked in" because there are witnesses (including yourself!) to your commitment. Start small (i.e., something commensurate with your fitness level, yet challenging at the same time); in other words, your first 5K should come before a 100-miler. Remember, several of our fitness friends from chapters 2 and 3 had no interest in racing until they got a taste of it.

Peer Pressure

Teenagers aren't the only ones who must contend with peer pressure. Although it takes on a different look — your drinking buddies (what, are you too good for us now) — smoking cronies (you'll be back) — your mother (have another piece of cake, Dear; I made it just for you; it's your favorite) — and your mate (you know *you could* build your muscles by fixing the screen door instead of wasting your time with that non-productive weightlifting) — will probably not be *totally* supportive. Being that friends and family are the mainstays of our lives (and are even important for maintaining our health), this is a huge hurdle to surmount. Many can never clear this obstacle.

The 60-Second Solutions will help. Beyond this, invite them to come with you on your new journey. They probably won't, but at least you didn't totally forsake them. You didn't leave them; *they* chose not to go with you. That's the best way to view it. And if they do decide to be a partner in renewal, wow! wouldn't that be wonderful? If not, try to see them under different circumstances where drinking, smoking, etc. is not on the agenda. Go places with them where the habit you've left behind takes a backseat to the activity at hand. With family, have a small piece of pie and don't commit to training and races during family time (e.g., Thanksgiving, Easter, Anniversaries, family suppertime, and the like).

The key is what you choose to focus upon. If you make your well-being a priority and you put your attention on activities that make you fitter, then all will work out well.

I'll Just Diet To Lose Weight

Exercise beats dieting for losing weight *and keeping it off.* In a study researchers divided participants into three groups: one group exercised and dieted; another only exercised; and the third only dieted. After two years, only the group that had exercised without dieting maintained its weight loss.

Losing weight by dieting depends on our depriving ourselves of foods that we would prefer to eat. Deprivation seldom works for very long, for obvious reasons. On the other hand, exercise doesn't deprive us of anything, but rather gives us something to do in place of eating all the time. Also, a good workout causes the release of endorphins into our system, which results in a pleasant exercise "high" — a good substitute for the pleasure of snacking on high-calorie foods.

Intense aerobic workouts and strength training cause the body's metabolism to rise, resulting in the burning of calories long after the exercise is over. Strength training has the additional benefit of building muscle, which burns fat 24 hours a day. One study of 15 sedentary individuals in their sixties and seventies found that after six months of weight training, they had increased their daily calorie burn by 230 and almost a third of this was from an increased metabolism.

Some think that if they exercise, they'll just eat more. British researchers at the University of Leeds studied the relationship of exercise/activity to appetite. After examining

32 studies, they found that active people ate just enough to replace the calories they burned. Some of the studies showed that couch potatoes ate about 500 more calories than their more vigorous peers. In the newest research, by the Dallas-based Cooper Institute's research team, 3-day diet records of more than 10,000 men and women were gathered and then these participants were given a state-of-the-art treadmill test to measure their fitness. The fit men consumed an average of 2,378 calories per day, while the unfit males averaged 30 more calories or 2,408. The unfit ladies devoured just 28 more calories, 1,887 to 1,859. One major difference between the eating habits of the fit versus the unfit was that the fit ate more carbohydrates in the form of fruits and vegetables, while the unfit downed more fat. It is obvious from these studies that exercising doesn't make us eat more, but it does cause one to eat a little better in many cases.

Low calorie diets can cause the body to "think" that there is a famine, and therefore, to slow the metabolism and hold onto fat until the crisis (dearth of food) has passed. It's apparent that diet alone is not the best way to go about losing weight *and keeping it off.* The best way to do that is to eat a healthy diet with only the occasional Hot Fudge Brownie Sundae and to exercise wisely; that is, do strength and aerobic training.

Not Inclined To Run 100 Miles or Climb Mt. Everest

Sherman Bull, a 64-year-old physician from New Canaan, Connecticut recently became the oldest person to climb Mount Everest (to the top). You may be saying, "Bully for him. I don't want to climb no stinkin' mountain." The good news is, you don't have to. The less fit you are, the less you have to do to become more fit. For some, a 20-minute walk several times a week would do them wonders. Others would need more of a challenge and probably would cherish it.

I Don't Like To Exercise

You don't have to. You can put on your favorite music and dance around the house. Another possibility for getting your exercise without "exercising" is to do housework at twice your normal speed for 10, 15, or 20 minutes at a time. Park at the farthest corner of the parking lot or garage and walk to the store or office. Take the steps instead of the elevator at least part of the way; walk a few flights up past your floor and then walk back down. Get a dog and take him for his daily walks. Chop logs for the fireplace, play tag with your grandkids, do knee bends and toe raises while talking on the phone, or take up a sport. In other words, put physical movement back into your everyday life. If it's fun, it's not really exercise — it's play! To stay young, make sure you play every day!

Costs Too Much

The truth is, it costs too much not to exercise. Researchers compared active folks (three or more moderate to strenuous 30-minute sessions or activities per week) who were fifteen and older to less active individuals and found that the exercised group saved $330 a year in doctors' visits, medication, and hospitalization. And the savings grew with age. Non-smoking men 45 and older who exercised saved $949. Those with health conditions that limited activity had to spend $1,053 more annually on medical costs. This study, done by the Centers for Disease Control and Prevention (CDC), reports that if all sedentary Americans became physically active, we could save $29.2 billion (1987 dollars) or $76.6 billion (2000 dollars) a year. You may be thinking that Medicare will cover these costs for you. According to the AARP Bulletin (October, 2001), Medicare at this time covers just over half of the healthcare expenses of enrollees as a whole; and the annual Part B premium is projected to climb from $600 in 2001 to $1,320 in 2011. Out-of-pocket expenses as a percentage of the senior's income is expected to rise, too.

On the other hand, the only cost for a basic exercise program is the expense of a comfortable pair of walking or running shoes. Or one could just dance around in his basement in his bare feet and do crunches/sit-ups and push-ups for free. Those opting for the more glamorous skiing and polo will find fitness takes a little more of an investment.

Rather Focus On Mental Activities

Chess World Champion Gary Kasparov is reported to exercise like an Olympic athlete in the months preceding a big match. There aren't too many activities more purely mental than chess.

136

The Mentalist, The Amazing Kreskin, as he travels around the country to amaze people, always takes a long walk around the local area first, followed by some serious stretching before each show.

The National Institute on Aging announces, "The good news is that most people can keep their mental capacities from declining just by doing things like *walking* [my emphasis], reading the newspaper, taking music class, ..."

Remember, the mind and the body work together as a team. The mind is the more important of the two, but without the body it has a hard time getting around.

A Single Parent Or Grandparent
If you are a single parent or grandparent (raising a grandchild) you know that time is not on your side. You'd like to exercise, but who has the time? One solution would be to get married. Short of that insane idea (just kidding, I think) here are some other options:

Get up a half hour early and do some form of exercise (stay in the house if there are young children involved). Take a 10 to 20-minute walk or run during lunch hour if you work outside the home. Play a game of basketball, soccer, tag, ... or skate, bike, ... with the kids after supper. Put your little tyke in a bike seat or jogging-stroller and off you go. Take the kids to the local high school track (with some toys) and run laps while they play on the infield. Use a treadmill, stationary bike, etc. while watching TV with them. Bottom line: although it's not always easy and takes some planning and time management skills, it is doable. Best of all, it will give you more energy (if done right) to deal with the harried life you live as both Mom and Dad to your children.

Well, there you have it. One excuse after another cut down in the prime of life. Any more excuses that you come up with you'll have to shoot down yourself or settle for a sluggish, rundown wreck of a body. The choice is yours.

CHAPTER 6 SUSTENANCE ABUSE

When did eating become so confounded complicated? There are low-fat diets, high-fat diets, high-protein/low-carbohydrate diets, and high-carbohydrate diets. As if that weren't enough, now we have to deal with saturated fats, polyunsaturated fats, monounsaturated fats, trans fats (or trans fatty acids), and even fake fats (for weight loss, which have no calories simply because the body doesn't know how to digest them). And where do omega 3, omega 6, and omega 9 fatty acids fit into this picture?

At one time it seemed like it was just a matter of getting our vitamin C, vitamin A, iron , and calcium. Remember that simpler time not so long ago? Now there's selenium for preventing asthma; folate or folic acid for birth defects; lutein for our eyes; lycopene for the prostate; quercetin for our hearts; potassium for high blood pressure; soluble fiber for our cholesterol; insoluble fiber for our bowels; AND lignans, glutathione, isoflavones, saponius, phytic acid, proteas inhibitors, indole-3-carbinol (13c for short), and sulforaphane for who knows what! And to make matters worse, scientists are hard at work finding new nutrients all the time!

Add to this the stuff that man adds to our foods: hydrolyzed corn protein, high-fructose corn syrup, autolyzed yeast extract, potassium sorbate, nitrates, nitrites, Aspartame, Sucrolose, yellow #5, and polysorbate 80. Yikes! We haven't even touched on genetically altered foods, irradiated foods, and preparation methods (i.e., deep fried versus broiled versus microwaved or "nuked" versus steamed versus stir fried versus raw).

Our hunter-gatherer ancestors didn't have such a mess with which to deal. They didn't have to worry about whether berries were better for them than bison burgers or whether to supplement their diet with succulent termite eggs (to get the folic acid missing from their diet).

They ate berries when they found them *because* they found them and meat when they got an animal (as opposed to the animal getting them). And they were thankful for whatever it was because the alternative was to go hungry! This simplified diet served them well. However, since they only lived to the grand old age of 29 or 30 (that's 5 or 6 in dog years) they didn't have to deal with what to eat to be fitter after 50. We do!

So here's our dilemma. What do we eat to be fitter after 50? What are the most important nutrients for us to consume: vitamin E, vitamin C, protein, complex carbohydrates, omega-3 fatty acids, zinc, iron, calcium, lycopene, water, oxygen, ...? Or does the answer reside in what we need to avoid? What are the most harmful nutrients/substances that we should eshew? Are caffein, nicotene, and other drugs public enemy number one? How about refined sugar, saturated fats, trans fatty acids, red dye #9, or Twinkies?

First, let's be thankful that we have so many choices to make. We can select from isles and isles of a wide variety of foods, drinks, and other substances for our nourishment.

What would be the most important nutrient for us to consume if we could only choose one? Would it be protein? Without sufficient protein we could not build and repair the cells of which we are made.

Would it be carbohydrates? We require carbs for the energy to run our body and it is the brain's only source of energy.

What about water? Our body (including the brain) is about 70% water. Without it we could only survive a couple of days.

How about oxygen? We need oxygen for all the chemical reactions that keep us alive and after all, we can only survive for a few short minutes without it.

The answer must be oxygen. Right? Actually we need *all* of these nutrients to survive and we would quickly perish without any of them. Therefore, this question about what is the primary nutrient is academic at best. But no, oxygen (nor any of the other nutrients) is not the correct answer. The answer is our thoughts. The thoughts that *nourish* us will determine whether we are fitter after 50 or not.

Let me explain. Thoughts that we entertain frequently can become our beliefs. Our beliefs about our self compose our self image. Our self image determines to a large degree what we do to ourselves — what we consume. For example, how does one treat a fine motor vehicle? If we owned a vintage Ford Mustang, would we put kerosene in the gas tank, molasses in the crank case, or Pepsi in the radiator? I think not! Treasuring our car and wanting it to continue to run or take us places in style, as well as desiring the pleasure of driving it, we would take good care of it.

Likewise, if we love and truly appreciate our body, we take care of it just like our car. Our thoughts about our body, our self, determines our self image. If our self image is one of awe and reverence for our mind/body then we are unlikely to pollute it with poisonous fumes, destructive liquids, and foods that would gum up the works.

One of my friends, a man named Virgil, is building a new house for his wife and two teenage youngsters. He works with computers during the day for a living and builds the home in the evenings. Typically, during the week Virgil will perform his carpentry from 5:00 P.M. to 2:00 A.M. with a short break for supper (no snacks). He will then be in bed by 3:00 and up again just three hours later at 6:00 in the morning. On Fridays he works on the house from about 5:00 P.M. through the night and all day Saturday, finishing up Saturday evening. He claims to wake up rested and ready for a new day each and every day. He never sleeps more than six hours; he doesn't believe you can catch up on lost sleep, so he doesn't try. He says that more than six hours of sleep a night makes him groggy. What's Virgil's secret? Does he have a super food supplement he takes? Is he on drugs? Does he have a phenomenal diet (or just a great mattress)? The simple answer is that Virgil loves working on his new home. He enjoys working with raw wood — the smell — the feel — the sense of accomplishment. He is having the time of his life laying floors and hanging doors. His diet consists of a wide variety of nutritionally sound foods (he tries to eat well) and because he is immersed in joyful thoughts, his body is able to take the raw ingredients he gives it and convert them into energy to work/play long hours at a time. Unknown to him, he is a creative genius when he is doing his woodworking; and when creative geniuses (artists, sculptors, composers, writers, scientists, woodworkers ...) are in their creative mode or zone or flow state they can go long periods without sleep, without getting tired. I will remind you again that our friend Helen Klein says that competing in multi-day races is "more mental than physical." We are nourished by our thoughts more than any food; but we do need the food, too.

Thoughts that create positive emotions and positive emotions that lead to positive, empowering thoughts put the body in an anabolic state (a building stage). Stress, negative thoughts, reflected in negative emotions, puts our body in a catabolic state where the flesh is broken down to create energy to fight or run away from the illusory "life-threatening" situation.

Imagine a fort in the old west with Indians (Native Americans) surrounding and attacking it. Under this situation, all those in the fort are going to discontinue their everyday tasks and put their energies into helping to keep the Indians from overrunning the place. Saving the fort from imminent destruction (and thus the inhabitants' demise) takes precedence. Washing clothes, fixing the hinges on the kitchen door, writing letters to friends back in Baltimore, and baking pies for the weekend festivities take a back seat. Taking ammunition and food to the soldiers and shoring up the fort's entrance doors replaces these everyday activities. Survival comes front and center.

A similar thing happens with your body under attack *or perceived attack.* Anger, fear, irritation, sadness (any "negative" emotion) signals the body that there is imminent danger. All is not well. Digestion of food, repair of cells, growth of new cells all take a backseat to survival. Blood is diverted from the stomach and other nonessential places to the arms and legs for battle. Cortisol is produced in the place of human growth hormone. Fighting pesky microorganisms is not as critical as saving the human being from the perceived life or death situation (perception is all). There is no need to digest food, fight minute microorganisms, or repair individual cells if the host body or organism is going to be dead in a few minutes, anyway, from an outside attack.

However, when the stressor is short-lived, there is no problem. Everything gets back to normal and digestion proceeds and microbes are escorted out of the body. But when stress becomes a normal state, a habitual state, the cells become battle weary, tissues don't get repaired, food doesn't get delivered to the cells, and toxic wastes build up and disposal becomes inefficient. Over time, tension interferes with the everyday activities of the body and the individual's well-being starts to decline.

When we stay primarily angry, depressed, or irritated for days or weeks at a time because our thoughts are focused on the negative side of life, the body and mind start to break down. On the flip side, staying joyful, excited, enthusiastic, or passionate about life allows the body/mind to heal and recreate itself during this time of peace. This is the body's version of what is called the peace dividend. During this state of positive thoughts and emotions the body/mind can use the raw materials (food and drink) to repair cells and build new ones.

If our thoughts (self-image) are of a body/mind that is sluggish, confused, fat, skinny, out of shape, and/or lacking energy, then we will find ourself eating a diet that supports this limiting image of ourself. If on the other hand, our self-image/thoughts are of an energetic, good looking, muscular, sexy, beautiful, and fit body, then we will find ourself consuming that which creates more of the same. For help with this mental-underpinning of a fitter you, see the mental exercises in chapter 4 and the 60-Second Solutions in chapter 7. Now let's turn our attention to what foods support a fit, healthy mind/body.

Fueling The Masters of Fitness
Let's review how eight of the Masters of Fitness fueled their awesome accomplishements. This will keep them, some of their accomplishments, and their dietary patterns fresh in our minds so that we can better see the relationship between them and the scientific data and ideas presented in this chapter.

Payton Jordan Chows Down ...
Here is a sampling of how Payton fueled his 12.0-second 100-meter world record at the Senior Olympics when he was 63. To put this in perspective, this is faster than 95% of college students and many college athletes could run it (my estimate).

Payton eats a simple diet with lots of vegetables and fruit. His meat intake is balanced equally between beef, lamb, pork, fish, and chicken. He's quoted as saying, "I'm a big fruit eater" and that "we [he and his family] eat few eggs and not much bacon or ham." Breakfast centers around oatmeal, Cream of Wheat, and sometimes dried cereals, such as shredded wheat and granola. Other items on his breakfast table include toast, orange juice, and cocoa. Lunch usually consists of cottage cheese, yogurt, and/or soup; and includes milk or hot tea as a beverage. I should mention that Payton does have a weakness for chocolate (but then, chocolate has gotten some good press lately).

Ruth Anderson Fuels With ...

Ruth, now in her early seventies, has held several national records and has over 70 ultra-marathons to her credit.

Ruth has this to say about her diet, "... my 'diet' [is] ... Not special, unless you call a typical runner's diet that much different or unusual. Pastas are high on the list of common food, but I do try to balance it with proteins, including red meat along with lots of fish and fowl. I am particularly fond of yogurt, fruit of all kinds and more selective on vegetables. Do drink beer and wine, mostly with meals, and love dark chocolate, to name a 'weakness' or two. I do like ethnic meals, especially in all the traveling I do."

On the food supplement front she adds, "I do take vitamins, and have for many years. Multi with fluoride for a while; C and E long before the good effects of E were reported; [and] dessicated liver, also early on for the extra iron content. Really do think I get enough of most of these in my diet, but feel travel and extra long running need greater 'support.' Haven't had a cold in years!"

Warren Utes' Diet

Warren has held around 70 national running records and at 81 is still going strong AND RACING!

Warren emphasizes fruits and vegetables in his diet and tries to eat "properly." He and his wife like stir-fried vegetables with tofu, limit the fat content of their meals, and drink plenty of fluids. Warren supplements his excellent eating habits with vitamin E and baby aspirin, but takes no other medicines.

Carl Kristenson Bulks Up With ...

Carl placed fifth in the Over-60 Mr. America bodybuilding contest. Carl eats to build muscle while limiting fat — a real "tightrope-walking act." His contest diet totals 1,800 calories per day and consists of egg whites, tuna, chicken, and salads (with vinegar topping). For fruit, Carl likes apples, bananas,

143

and raisins, but he has to be careful to limit his fruit so that his total calories don't exceed his 1,800 quota. His grains are whole grains in the form of whole wheat bread and oatmeal. He tries to drink eight glasses of water a day, but has trouble doing this; he likes his black coffee a little too much. In order to bulk up, he eats a lot of protein as you can see. He is a steroid-free, all-natural bodybuilder, but does use some over-the-counter body-building supplements found at health food stores like GNC.

June Tatro Eats Well

June is our 87-year-old fitness instructor, ballroom dancer, and part-time contortionist.

June considers diet as a very essential component of fitness and good health. She is a proponent of the upside down nutrition pyramid and eats accordingly. At the top and the widest part of this pyramid are vegetables (which make up the largest percentage of her diet). Then comes fruit; followed by whole grains; and then dairy, fish, meats, fats/oils, and an ocassional sweet (junk food) — in that order.

When it comes to supplements, she says that "everyone has a different system and can't take this or that." Therefore, she strongly suggests that one get a qualified health professional to recommend a good multi-vitamin (which should contain folic acid, among other ingredients). June would probably want me to tell you that the reason seniors need supplemental vitamins is because the older we get, the less able we are to efficiently absorb vitamins, minerals, and other nutrients — unless we have taken very good care of ourselves.

James Hill's Morsels For Marathons

James went from an overweight, sedentary typical middle-aged American to an American marathon champion in about seven years. Here is the diet that fueled this metamorphosis:

Each morning for about 10 years now, James has filled a blender with three bananas and orange juice for an ample breakfast smoothie (a mega-potassium, blood-pressure-friendly drink). At lunch, a normal meal for James would be a serving of fish or barbecued meat, pinto beans and cole slaw. Once a week he eats at a cafeteria where he will typically have three servings of vegetables, salad and bread (no meat). He does not eat dessert at noon. His evening meal is usually smaller and often consists of just mixed fruit or soup. An after supper dessert of jello or ice cream is common. James often eats an orange, apple or banana in the evening or some other time during the day. He seldoms eats what he considers to be "fast foods" and has been taking a multi-vitamin for about a year as nutritional insurance. We will address his generous fluid intake later in this chapter.

Jerry Dunn — America's Marathon Man Fuels Up

Jerry's latest ultra-challenge was running 200 marathons in 2000 at the age of 54. Here's where he gets the energy to accomplish such incredible feats of endurance.

Jerry attempts to eat five or six times per day — small portions. Typically his day looks like this: For breakfast he has oatmeal with a banana, brown sugar and milk on it, and orange juice. His mid-morning snack is a Power Bar (high-protein bar) and water. Lunch is tuna, beef or chicken with a salad, bread, water and sometimes apple pie. An afternoon snack usually consists of a fruit smoothie with Endurox R4 (an electrolyte, glycogen, ... replacement drink powder). Supper consists of pork, chicken, beef or fish with corn, green beans, bread and water. For his evening snack he often turns to salted popcorn, an apple and cheese.

In the supplement department, Jerry has been using Barley Essence from Green Foods (liquid greens) since March, 1993. Jerry sees the B E helping him "... maintain a high level of energy; fight inflammation (from overuse of muscles, ...); and supply the 'greens' [he needs] in his diet." And as you read, he also takes a potent Gatorade-type drink — Endurox R4. In 2001 he added glucosamine/chondroitin for stiffness in his knees (200 marathons in one year will do that to some folks).

During marathons Jerry drinks plenty of water and Endurox R4 for his high fluid needs. For energy, he turns to packets of Power Gel (an energy replacement product), bananas, and an occasional coffee and glazed donut.

Woman Athlete of the "Century's" Nutritional Foundation

In 1995, at the age of 72, Helen Klein completed the grueling 145-mile Marathon Des Sables — a multi-day race across the Sahara Desert (and adjoining, similarly brutal terrain) in Morocco; just two weeks later she took on and finished the first Eco-Challenge (a 370-mile multi-sport race (horseback riding, rock climbing, canoeing, ...). Where did Helen get the energy and awe-inspiring recuperative powers? Much of it came from her mindset, but without adequate, proper nutrition, no amount of mental magic or positive thinking could get her the first 25 miles, never mind the rest.

Helen eats a wide variety of healthful foods from whole grains to a variety of high-protein sources. But her diet centers around the mega-consumption of fruits and vegetables. Specifically, she puts away 5 or 6 fruits AND 5or 6 vegetables each day. Her diet also includes a daily 4-ounce helping of ham, steak or chicken (all fat trimmed). Most of Helen's meals are home cooked and she stays away from "fast foods" and sodas. However, during long-distance competitions she will down sodas for the caffein needed to stay awake and alert. She does partake of coffee in the morning and tea throughout the day. Interestingly, in very recent studies, tea, both green and black, has been shown to be a boon to our health. One of Helen's favorite foods is apples (and we know what an apple a day keeps away).

The day before an ultra race Helen "eats huge amounts of pasta, fruit, and veggies." During a long-distance race she will sometimes need as many as 8,000 calories per day just to maintain and resupply her 109 to 112-pound frame.

She had never taken any food supplements, not even a multi-vitamin, until Kenneth Cooper, M.D., of the Cooper Aerobic Institute talked her into taking antioxidants when she was 75.

What To Eat To Be Fitter After 50

What can we glean from our Masters of Fitness concerning what to eat? They are certainly leading by example; no cheap talk here. If these FA50 role models can perform as well as they do and accomplish such Herculean feats, then maybe we can adopt some of their eating habits and strategies so as to have the energy, fitness and health required for living our everyday lives to the fullest. Their diets are all different, but there are some similarities, and we can come to some general conclusions.

Veggies Reign Supreme

Mom was right when she insisted, "Eat your vegetables, Dear!" At the same time, she couldn't know just how right she was. Yes, she knew about tomatoes for vitamin C, carrots for vitamin A, and vegetables in general for "your vitamins and minerals, Sweetheart." But since that time when she coaxed you to open up and let the make-believe food-bumblebee "buzz-buzzzzz" down your gullet or warned you that there would be "no dessert" or "no going out to play with your friends" until the dreaded vegetables were "down the hatch," the scientists have discovered a thing or two.

These vegetable detectives with their white lab coats have discovered that potassium helps lower blood pressure and is found in abundance in beans, avocados, potatoes, celery and lima beans, as well as steamed clams, bananas and apricots. Let's take a closer look at this.

High blood pressure plagues a third of all Americans in their fifties, half of those in their sixties and fully two thirds of the over-seventy crowd. It puts 50 million older Americans at risk of strokes, heart attacks and kidney failure. Yet, the people of non-industrialized countries do not share this pattern of blood pressure increasing with age; whether they reside in China, Africa, Alaska or the Amazon, individuals in more primitive settings experience no age-related change in blood pressure.

According to Dr. Paul Whelton of Tulane University, the reason is very simple: people in primitive cultures do not eat processed food. Dr. Whelton spent a decade tracking 15,000 indigenous Yi people of China. As long as they subsisted on their traditional diet, abundant in rice, fruits and *vegetables*, these rural farmers hardly ever developed hypertension. But those that moved to nearby towns were found to have blood pressures that began to rise with age.

Some researchers think this is due in part to the increased salt content of many processed foods, such as "fast foods," canned foods, frozen dinners, pretzels, ... For example, a 4-ounce tomato contains just 9 mg. of sodium, whereas a 4-ounce can of tomato sauce has 700 mg. For tens of thousands of years man's food has had a potassium-to-sodium ratio of 10 to 1. In the last 50 years or so, with the advent and consumption of processed foods, the average twenty-first century American consumes a diet that has more sodium than potassium.

Scientists have found that a daily diet low in fat with ten servings of fresh or frozen fruits and *vegetables* (such as Helen Klein's diet) and two servings of low-fat dairy (for calcium) is very effective in lowering blood pressure and keeping it at healthy levels.

Another vegetable that helps with stabilizing one's blood pressure is celery, but not for the potassium content (as we might expect). When scientists studied celery they found that it contains a chemical compound called 3-n-butyl phthalide that lowers blood pressure an average of 12 to 14 percent in lab animals. This compound, with the big name, was discovered to relax the muscles of the arteries and to reduce stress hormone levels, thus reducing the constriction of the blood vessels (blood pressure is increased when blood vessels are constricted).

Now let's turn our attention from vegetables for stabilizing blood pressure to vegetables as a source of calcium. In places around the world, such as rural China where dairy products are sparse, people get their calcium from eating dark leafy greens like kale, dandelion and turnip (these, of course, are the North American versions of the greens). For example, a single helping of kale supplies 8 percent of the U.S. RDA (Recommended Daily Allowance) for calcium and is particularly well absorbed. Other greens, such as spinach, collards, beet and swiss chard are loaded with oxalates that interfere with the complete absorption of calcium, but they are jam-packed with other advantageous nutrients. As a matter of fact, greens pack the most nutrients per calorie of any food. As an illustration, a helping of collards or kale is only 30 calories and supplies 8% of the RDA for calcium and countless other nutrients; while sharp cheddar cheese and 2% milk have 110 and 130 calories respectively and supply 30% of the RDA for calcium and fewer other nutrients.

Another group of vegetables that is hard to beat is the cruciferous family. Its family members include broccoli, cabbage, kale, turnip, cauliflower, brussel sprouts, and bok choy. Among a multitude of other nutrients, they contain sulfuraphane, which is thought to protect against cancer. New studies at Johns Hopkins University and Tsukuba University in

Japan show that the cruciferous vegetables also contain phase II enzymes that actually detoxify cancer-causing agents before they can be activated to do damage to cells which can lead to cancer. The crucifers also help lower cholesterol, improve heart health, prevent constipation, strengthen the immune system, preserve eyesight and dial 911 in case of an emergency. You get the picture. They, along with dark leafy greens, are very good for us, and the average American only ingests about one-quarter of a cup of these health and fitness enhancers on a given day.

But that's not all! Carrots, sweet potatoes, pumpkins, mangoes and apricots (the orange gang) are overflowing with beta carotene, which preserves eyesight, strengthens the immune system, supports heart health, prevents memory loss, and helps with arthritis and diabetes, to name a few benefits. Chile peppers have capsaicin, a phyto-nutrient that helps regulate blood clots. Zucchini and orange peppers preserve eyesight due to their secret ingredient, zeaxanthin.

A geneticist at the Agricultural Research Service of the United States Department of Agriculture recently discovered eight flavonoids in the bean coat (you know, the one that keeps a bean warm on a cold winter's night). Flavonoids are colored pigments that may be the antioxidant/protective factor in red wine and other foods. Antioxidants neutralize free radicals before they can do damage to our cells, and thus cause us to age. Six of the eight newly-discovered flavonoids that were found in the above-mentioned bean coat were particularly strong antioxidants.

Who can keep up with all of this? Not I. The good news is, we don't need to. All we need to do is follow the lead of James, Jerry, Helen, June and Payton and eat several servings a day of a wide variety of vegetables.

Fruit, Fruit, And More Fruit

Momma was right *again* when she told you that, "Fruit is good for you. Have another helping, Honey." What do all our Masters of Fitness have in common, besides eating a ton of vegetables? They followed Mom's advice and loaded up on fresh fruit.

The question is: What do fruits have to offer us besides their variety of delicious, naturally sweet (and tart) tastes? Like

149

vegetables, they are loaded with fiber, and some recent research has found that those who eat plenty of fiber stay slender even if they pay little attention to the rest of their diet. One study found that individuals with type II diabetes who ate a high fiber diet (50 grams per day) not only lowered their cholesterol, but also their blood-sugar level.

Many fruits are loaded with antioxidants that do battle with cell-destroying free radicals that have racked up countless frequent flyer miles traveling coast to coast inside your skin. For example, a study of 40 fruits and vegetables found that blueberries (a fruit) surpassed them all in antioxidant power because they are loaded with the same anthocyanins that have given red wine its reputation as a free-radical scavenger. Red grapes, cherries and plums also contain this super-duper antioxidant, as do strawberries, red raspberries and currants. But the media would rather promote the antioxidant properties of wine (it's "cooler" — more "hip") than the benefits of grape juice (or blueberries on your cereal) to fight heart disease, protect vision and tame cancer.

Lycopene, a component of tomatoes, has hit the country's top-40 billboard of nutrients, but did you know that the red coloring of lycopene tells you that it is also in pink grapefruit and watermelon? We know to eat or drink citrus fruits (especially orange juice) to get ample vitamin C, but do we know anything else about oranges and their cousins? For instance, tangerines contain beta-cryptoxanthin, which transforms into vitamin A in our body. Two other compounds in tangerines are tangeretin and nobiletin, which appear to prevent breast cancer; leukemia researchers at the University of Western Ontario in London, Canada found them to be 250 times more powerful than the mighty-and-much-publicized soybean's phytochemical, genistein, formerly the poster boy of anti-cancer phytonutrients. But before you run out and corner the market on tangerines, you should know that grapefruit, strawberries, blackberries, blueberries, raspberries and pomegranates all contain substantial amounts of ellagic acid (a polyphenol), an antioxidant that is known to slay tumors.

Let us not forget that the flavonoids in cranberries help prevent urinary tract infections in elderly women and help prevent low-density (LDL — "the bad") cholesterol from becoming oxidized. Oxidized LDL is much more likely to find its way to the arterial walls to form dangerous plaques. But before you scurry off to bag a bushel of cranberries, know that each fruit (and vegetable) has its own story to tell concerning how it is better than Mighty Mouse for saving the day and our health.

Again, one of the secrets to the fountain of youth that Warren, James and Ruth have apparently found is to frequently eat a wide variety of fresh and frozen fruits (I recommend thawing first). We can't go wrong unless they are buried inside a refined-sugar-laden pie or stuffed in the recesses of a grape-jelly donut (save these mouth-watering, blood-sugar-spiking desserts for savoring on special/limited occasions — we will enjoy them all the more because we haven't overdosed on them on a regular basis).

Clean Your Plate, Dear

Mommy was right when she told us to eat our fruits and vegetables, but when it came to portions — whoops! "Finish your dinner; clean your plate; and remember the starving Armenians." Remember those admonitions or ones similar to them? Cleaning our plate when we were children, whether we were hungry or not, for many of us became a lifelong habit. As an adult, it turned into cleaning our plate after second and third helpings whether we needed the food or not. We seem to have taken Mom's counsel to heart, resulting in one who doesn't listen to his own body when it says, "Whoa, Miss Piggy!" The child who dutifully cleaned his plate has become the grown-up who eats too much of the wrong stuff and even too much of the right stuff (nutritious foods).

As a result (in part), from 50 to 61 percent of adult Americans are said to be overweight or obese depending on what criterion is used and which study is cited. Whatever the actual figure is, it's obvious that America is an "XXL" nation and getting bigger.

There are several factors which, when taken together, add up to a big, fat problem. There's the sedentary factor. That is, TV watching, computer gazing, ... Along this line, there are satellite communities on the fringes of our cities that discourage walking, biking and such due to a lack of sidewalks and biking/hiking trails, and a plethora of pedestrian-unfriendly roadways. Foodwise we are surrounded by

151

temptation — delicious high-fat, high-sugar, hi-big-fat-thighs-and-bellies foods. Then there's the issue at hand (remember), portion sizes.

Foreign visitors to our soil are amazed by two things: how large our food servings are and how big and fat Americans are. Could there be a relationship here? A cause and effect correlation? The United States Department of Agriculture's figures show that we are consuming on average 148 more calories per day than we were just twenty years ago. That can add up to several additional pounds of blubber each year if we don't take some preventive action.

Here are some examples of how we Americans tend to blow things out of pro*portion,* so to speak. In France, the croissant contains 174 calories and 11 grams of fat; the "same" croissant here in the U.S. of A. has grown to 270 calories and 15 grams of fat. Poland's bagels have 116 calories and weigh about 1.5 ounces; the American version balloons to 4.5 ounces with a whopping 350 calories. The quesadilla of Mexico weighs in at 540 calories and 32 grams of fat; here in America our rendition swells to 1,200 calories and 70 grams of fat. We must think bigger is better: bigger hips, bigger bellies and bigger buttocks.

According to *Environmental Nutrition,* September, 2000, a regular hamburger, small fries and a small drink in a typical fast-food restaurant (the size nobody gets) has about 600 calories. Upgrading (interesting terminology) this dinner to a "value meal" doubles its calorie content. "Supersizing" it can put this meal at about 1,800 calories. That means that almost a full day's recommended quota of calories is downed at a single meal (or in many cases as a between meal snack) and without a single serving of fruits and vegetables (unless you want to count fat-drenched french fries as a vegetable). No wonder a study at Purdue University found that there was a strong correlation between frequent eating out at restaurants and a high or "unhealthy" body mass index (a measure of one's height-to-weight ratio or obesity).

What can we do short of leaving the country for distant, slender shores or stopping eating out? We can order the smaller-size menu offerings or cut our servings in half when we first get them and put one half in a "doggy bag" right away to preclude temptation. As we mentioned, Helen Klein cuts her meat and fish into 4-ounce servings, trims the fat, and eats almost all her meals at home or eats as close to "home-cooking" as she can when she's on the road. All our Masters of Fitness eat moderate and small portions except when they are carbohydrate loading for a big race or loading up on muscle-building protein in preparation for a body-building competition as in Carl's case. Skipping dessert or sharing one with our dinner partner is another option. Of course, eating more meals at home or brown-bagging it are possibilities, too. When at home, we can slice the entree and place it on our plate rather than bringing the whole lasagna dish to the table. This cuts down on our temptation to keep digging out more and more lasagna (or roast beast, ...) and piling it on our plate. Just make a decision before the meal starts to have only one serving. We may find that the only thing we need to do to lose weight and keep it off is to eat smaller portions (and get some exercise, of course). That way we don't have to deny ourselves anything that we like. Deprivation seldom works for long. By eating slower and savoring each mouthful more, we won't even notice that we are eating less. Therefore, we won't feel the deprivation of anything (other than a few inches around our waist).

Frequent, Small Meals

Sumo wrestlers (you know, the big, big guys with the "pants" that look like thong diapers) usually eat only two meals per day so as to put on weight. Individuals trying to diet often skip meals and eat so little during the day that they become ravenous at night. Not able to resist, they end up bingeing after a couple of days or so of deprivation and denial. You wouldn't know anyone like that, would you?

On the other hand, male fitness contestants and bodybuilders with well-defined muscle, percentage of body fat in the *single digits* (the average for the typical American male is 23% [the ideal is around 15%] and for the women it is 32 [ideal about 22]) and small, almost nonexistent waists eat 5 to 7 small meals a day. Bill Phillips' Million Dollar Body-For-Life Fitness Challenge, which has helped tens of thousands of individuals just like you and me lower their percentage of body fat dramatically and drop unwanted inches, recommends eating six meals a day. From the above examples,which do you think works better, starving all day and then eating one large meal in the evening or eating several smaller meals throughout the day?

Eating huge meals can slow our metabolism and make us feel sluggish (think Thanksgiving, when the turkey isn't the only thing that gets stuffed). The body doesn't need all the carbohydrates and fats consumed at a large repast to meet its calorie requirements — its energy needs. Therefore, when the glycogen stores in the liver and muscles are full, the excess carbs and surplus fat are deposited as fat on our hips, belly and elsewhere until we need it for energy (which might be never). Since the liver and muscles only hold 200 to 500 total grams of glycogen, it doesn't take too many big meals to make a big belly. Fat storage, unlike glycogen, is infinite. This accounts for the ocassional news story of the two-ton person who has to have the side of his house removed to get him to the hospital. We could run for days, hundreds of miles (some say from Florida to New York, for example), on our stored fat, but marathoners "hit the wall" (i.e., run out of glycogen) at about the 20-mile mark if they haven't replenished it at aid stations along the way.

To be a member of the National Weight Control Registry, one has to have lost at least 30 pounds and kept it off for a year or more. These individuals are our real weight-loss experts. They claim (and there are hundreds of them) that one of their most beneficial tactics for successfully controlling their weight is to eat an average of five times per day.

Eating 5 or 6 times a day is not as radical as it sounds. Many of us eat 3 meals each day with a mid-morning, mid-afternoon and evening snack; that's six feedings. To transform these feedings into six meals, just make the meals a little smaller and the snacks a little larger and more nutritious. Each mini-meal needs to be a balance of protein, carbohydrate (complex and simple), and some healthy fat. This takes preplanning, otherwise we end up eating junky snacks again. This means preparing some of our meals ahead of time and taking them with us if we will be out of the home during that day.

By eating frequently we don't get hungry and end up eating whatever is available: a candy bar, a piece of pie, a soda, or bingeing at night because we are so ravenous. Also, eating many balanced meals a day keeps our blood sugar stabilized so it doesn't fluctuate wildly, causing us problems and triggering hunger pangs. During ultra challenges Ruth, Jerry and Helen eat hour-by-hour to keep going — constant small feedings.

Small, frequent feedings is not the answer for everyone. A good example of this is Masters champion Nolan Shaheed, 52. This year Nolan broke five 50-plus world records: indoor 800 meters, 2:02.88; indoor mile, 4:27.14; indoor 3,000 meters, 8:54.73; road 5-k, 15:36; and outdoor 1,500 meters, 4:06.36. He did all this while eating just six meals a week (one after each workout); on the seventh day he rests, neither eating nor running. He claims that he is never hungry and always has plenty of energy (apparently so). Nolan is also an accomplished musician and composer and probably, as with many creative geniuses, doesn't need a lot of food or rest because he loves and gets "lost in" what he does.

The Insulin Factor

Getting fitter and healthier depends on keeping one's hormones in balance by living a healthy lifestyle. Let's take a look at the fuel-regulating hormone, insulin. Its job, along with glucogen, is to regulate sugar levels in our blood so that they don't get dangerously high or low. These two hormones are the master controllers of our metabolism. According to Dr. Jeffry Life, researcher and professor of nutrition science at Marywood University, 80 to 90 percent of the regulation of our blood sugar levels is the result of what we eat and the rest is exercise related.

When sugar levels in the blood are high, insulin is released to bring the amount of sugar (glucose) back to a safe level. Sugar burning as an energy source takes priority and fat is stored for later use; meanwhile, triglycerides and cholesterol in the blood can rise to "unhealthy levels." Chronically-elevated insulin levels is now seen as a major player in causing obesity, frequent food cravings and bingeing, mood swings, heart disease, and other chronic diseases.

Two things can cause insulin levels in our blood to rise to high levels, which, if continued over time, can cause problems:

    1. Carbohydrate consumption (especially those with an abundance of simple sugars)

155

2. Large meals (abundant carbohydrates and/or protein eaten at one sitting)

The solution is to eat 5 or 6 mini-meals each day with a balance of protein, carbohydrates (mostly complex and some simple) and healthful fats. Let's take a look at why we need a balance of the three macro-nutrients at each meal.

Protein

Somewhere along the line, protein became controversial, as in high-protein (and low-protein) diets. Keep in mind that there are only three macro-nutrients (carbohydrates, fats and proteins) that supply all our energy needs (calories). Vitamins, minerals and phytonutrients are all micro-nutrients that are needed in minute amounts (thus the "micro" label), but supply virtually no calories. Therefore, no matter how we combine the proteins, carbs and fats in our diet, they must total 100 percent of our calories consumed. For example, 65-percent carbs, 25-percent fat, and 10-percent protein is one of many possible combinations adding up to 100 percent. So in the end, all the controversy and name calling comes down to merely what percentage of our diet each macro-nutrient will be. How much protein do we need? What perentage would be best for us? First, let's take a closer look at protein and its role.

Other than water (which composes about 70 percent of our body), protein is the main component of the trillions of cells that collectively are us. To build and repair our cells, which we must do to stay healthy, "young," and vital, we need protein. Our enzymes that catalyze all bodily functions; our hormones which include the human growth hormone, testosterone, estrogen and insulin; and our immunoglobulins (the immune system) are all made of protein (and fatty acids). Our muscles are mostly *protein* and water. When our muscles atrophy from disuse and lack of protein we become frail and feeble. This unnatural shriveling of the muscles (and increase in fat) is often mistaken for old age. It is viewed as the natural aging process by most of us, instead of the disorder that it is.

Obviously we need protein. Can we get too much? Sure can. Can we get too little? Sure can. So how much protein should we consume?

Our hunter/gatherer, ancient ancestors ate a lot of protein in the form of meat (and we don't hear them complaining). More recently the Eskimos of Greenland, Alaska and Canada, for thousands of years, prospered on a diet comprised of fish, other marine animals and reindeer. This is what we would definitely call a high-protein/low-carbohydrate diet. Yet, until civilization reached them, bringing refined food products (high carb), disease, and tooth decay, they lived to a ripe old age — with little obesity, diabetes or cardiovascular disease.

Our own ancestors on the frontier in the 1800's ate a high percentage of fish, meat and eggs. Yet, heart disease was so rare that the first study of cardiovascular disease wasn't published in a medical journal until 1912 (yes, there were medical journals back then, but Brokaw just didn't broadcast their findings).

Now let's take a look at what our modern-day scientists are saying about protein. Some experts would argue that the recommended daily allowance (RDA) for protein is set for encouraging adequate consumption, not optimum intake for a super fit individual. Even so, a recent United States Department of Agriculture (USDA) study found that older individuals, and women in particular, are not meeting the minimum standard for protein intake. Specifically, 25 percent of men and 30 percent of women do not get enough protein in their diet; and it gets worse for older Americans, with 36 percent of men and 43 percent of women over the age of 70 being deficient. Also, when one is exercising vigorously, he or she needs even more protein to build and keep muscles strong, among other things.

A study cited in the American Journal of Nutrition showed the difference the percentage of protein to carbohydrate makes. They compared a diet that had a protein-to-carb ratio of .6 with one that had a ratio of .25 (such as the diet recommended by the American Heart Association). The .6 diet reduced the insulin response and had a positive nitrogen balance. In layman's terms, it promoted muscle development and discouraged the accumulation of fat stores; the .25 program did just the opposite, which means packing on pounds of fat and destroying muscle.

Another study, from Arizona State University, compared two diets: a 60 percent carbs, 25 percent fat and 15 percent protein version and a 30 percent carbs, 30 percent fat and 40 percent protein rendition. These scientists found that the higher protein diet caused the subjects to burn 58 more calories during the first 30 minutes after a meal.

Finally, Dr. Layman and associates at the University of Illinois compared the effects of changing the ratio of protein to carbohydrate in two 1,700-calorie-per-day diets. One group followed a 40 percent carbs, 30 percent fat and 30 percent protein protocol; the other observed federal dietary guidelines — 60 percent carbs, 30 percent fat and 10 percent protein. After ten weeks, both groups had lost an average of 16 pounds. The important distinction was *what* they actually lost. The high-protein group lost 12.3 pounds of body fat and just 1.7 pounds of muscle; while the lower-protein (federal guidelines) subjects dropped 10.4 pounds of fat and 3 pounds of muscle. I realize that the numbers don't add up to 16 pounds; so the rest of the loss must have been water. The point is, the higher protein consumption prevented the loss of lean muscle mass. In addition, the high-protein group increased its HDL (good guys) to LDL cholesterol ratio, decreased the triglycerides (fat) in the blood, and upped the thyroid hormone levels significantly (faster metabolism). Furthermore, the subjects reported being less hungry between meals and more energetic.

I know you're probably wondering how much protein you should eat. This depends on several factors, such as how active you are, how much muscle you want, your body type, etc. I recommend that you have a protein source with each of your 5 or 6 mini-meals. It could be fish, lean meat, peanut butter, tofu, high-protein veggie burgers, eggs, legumes, a dairy product (such as yogurt), or seeds and nuts.

Carbohydrates

There are two kinds of carbohydrates, simple and complex. The simple carbohydrates are the sugars found mostly in fruits, milk, and refined-sugar foods, such as candy, soda, desserts and of course, the sugar bowl. The complex carbohydrates are starches, found in abundance in rice, yams, potatoes, oatmeal, whole-grain breads, muffins, ...; and fiber, which is part-and-parcel of fruits, vegetables, nuts, and whole-grain products (i.e., all the food stuff derived from plants).

Scientists/nutritionists have developed a glycemic index which ranks foods by how much they affect our blood sugar levels. As we will see in the section on fat, blood sugar levels (especially sudden spikes in it) and the insulin response are closely related to fat storage, cardiovascular disease, and type II diabetes. This glycemic-index system can help us select foods that will keep our blood sugar levels stabilized. Many people swear by it and many more swear at it. It's complicated and requires one to memorize the GI ranking or value (satisfactory or unsatisfactory) or carry a card with the GI rankings of endless foods. Our fitness champions don't carry a GI card around with them. As a matter of fact, none of them even mentioned it, but it is worth a gander all the same.

The reason it is so frustrating is its unpredictability. For example, most candy is high glycemic and causes one's blood glucose to skyrocket, but Snickers candy bars don't, due to the ingredients: peanuts and dairy. Old-fashioned oatmeal is low glycemic, but instant and quick-cooking versions are intermediate glycemic. White bread is borderline high glycemic while spaghetti (made from coarser seminola flour) is low. Baked potatoes are high and sweet potaatoes are low. Most fruits are low, but pineapple is intermediate and dried dates are almost off the charts — high.

The advice from GI expert Jennie Brand-Miller, Ph.D., University of Sydney, Australia is to include at least one low-GI food as part of each snack or meal. Most fresh and frozen fruits, vegetables, and whole grains are low or intermediate glycemic. Therefore, when we load up on a wide variety of these staples, as our Masters of Fitness do, we will get a good glycemic balance. As a result, our all-important blood-sugar levels will be stabilized. Along with these fitness-producing foods (fruits, veggies, and whole grains) each meal/snack should include a high-protein food, some good fat, and a sturdy, complex carbohydrate, such as sweet potatoes, whole grain rice, oatmeal, etc. As with Jerry, Helen and James, one of the top secrets is to greatly limit our intake of high-glycemic sodas, candies and desserts.

Thermogenesis

Yet another method of selecting healthful foods for a fitter you involves thermogenesis. The thermogenic effect of foods refers to how many calories the body expends in the digestion and assimilation of a food. Any calories used up in the eating/metabolizing of a foodstuff cannot be added to our hips and belly as fat. For example, a serving of broccoli (according to the label on a box of broccoli in my freezer) has only 4 grams of carbohydrates, 2 of which are fiber (the thermogenic part of carbs). When we subtract 2 grams of fiber from 4 total grams of carbohydrates we get just 2 grams of active carbohydrates that could end up draped around our hips as body fat. Therefore, the number of calories available to the body for energy and/or storage as fat is even less than the mere 25 calories per serving noted on the label.

The thermogenic effect of different foods and individual metabolisms ranges from 10% to 35%. Consuming protein in the form of lean meat uses up about 30% of the calories; that is, if the piece of meat is labeled as having 200 calories, subtract 60 (30%) and you actually only end up consuming 140 calories. Carbs are medium thermogenic at 15% and fat has the lowest thermic value, 10%.

When it comes to carbs, high-water/high-fiber content (non-starch) fruits and vegetables have a high thermic-to-carbohydrate ratio. They are nutrient dense and calorie sparse and therefore can be eaten in almost unlimited amounts without adding poundage to our carcass. These highly recommended, very nutritious fruits and veggies include fresh and frozen: grapes, peaches, pears, raspberries, strawberries, apples, apricots, asparagus, blueberries, broccoli, cabbage, celery, cherries, lettuce, mushrooms, onions, radishes and spinach. Of course, if the broccoli is floating in a sea of butter or drowning in calorific sauces, then it loses its plethora-of-nutrients-in-a-handful-of-calories advantage.

Those with a less suitable thermic to carbohydrate ratio are: bananas, dates, figs, potatoes, yams, watermelon, and raisins and other dried fruits. These are all good foods to eat, but just not on such an unlimited basis since they are more carbohydrate dense/calorie loaded.

The carbs to avoid or at least limit are the nutrient-sparse/carbohydrate-dense/low-thermogenic refined white flour and sugar-processed foods, such as: sodas, cookies, cakes, pies, crackers, breads, muffins, ... Their high-calorie, low-nutrient characteristics make them a poor value even — especially if — they are labeled low fat or non-fat. For when the fat is taken out, the sugar, high-fructose corn syrup, etc. goes in to keep the product somewhat palatable. As the manufacturers sneak "sugar," little by little, into our foods under various aliases, we end up eating more and more nutrient-sparse/sugar-dense foods. These white flour breads and muffins are not to be confused with their nutrient-dense, whole-grain cousins.

As of 1999, the daily consumption of processed sugar in the U.S. had reached a staggering, blood-sugar-spiking, body-fat-storing 60 teaspoons per day for every man, woman and child in our great big, button-popping country. The American Journal of Clinical Nutrition recently stated that the average adult gets 27 percent of his daily calories from junk food. As we've seen, our fitness champions don't!

Fat Burns Fat

For over 20 years Americans have been encouraged by the "experts" to eat a low-fat diet; so in the ensuing years we have dutifully reduced our fat intake significantly (from around forty percent of our total calories to the lower thirties). What is our reward for these years of *sacrifice and deprivation*? We are fatter than ever and heart disease, cancer and other chronic diseases are still rampant. Despite leading the world in medical technology, we are mired at the bottom of the international rankings when it comes to obesity and the rate of degenerative diseases.

Meanwhile, the inhabitants of the Mediterranean island of Crete have one of the lowest incidences of heart disease while consuming 40 to 45 percent of their calories in the form of fat. Before they became westernized, Eskimos had a fat-laden meat and fish diet, but very little obesity or cardiovascular risk. What's going on here?

Let's switch gears and look at a single individual and his fat intake. A couple of years ago, Jim Morris won the Masters Olympia bodybuilding contest for men 60 and older. His chiseled, 5-foot, 9-inch, 210-pound body shows not a hint of a fat corpuscle anywhere. He looks better built than 99.9 percent of the young stud bodybuilders one would see at the local gym. In an article in Modern Maturity magazine, he attributes his awesome physical presence to his daily fitness routine and his diet. Specifically, he starts off by saying , "I eat a lot of peanuts. In the shell, unsalted. I sit and shell peanuts and have a bit of fruit." Peanuts are 70% fat and yet, according to this magazine interview, they are a centerpiece of his diet.

Now listen to this. Prevention Magazine came out with the Amazing Peanut Butter Diet in 2000. That's right, a diet centered around fat-oozing peanut butter. This diet is based on the research of Kathy McManus, R.D., at Brigham Women's Hospital in Boston. One hundred and one overweight women were divided into two groups; one followed a 20% fat diet and the other followed a 35% monounsaturated fat diet (including nuts, olive oil, avocados and, of course PB). The calories were the same for both groups: 1200 for women and 1500 for men. The participants in each group lost about 11 pounds in the first six weeks; but twice as many "peanut butter" dieters stuck with their diet and maintained their losses for 18 months. Those in the low-fat group that stuck it out regained an average of 5 pounds. Why? It is easier to stick with a diet that includes a modicum of fat because it cuts cravings and satisfies the desire for some tasty foods, while depriving one's self is always an uphill battle.

And just as interesting were the health benefits. The diet rich in monounsaturated fats was just as successful at lowering total cholesterol and the "bad" LDL cholesterol as was the low-fat fare. In addition, the "peanut butter" diet *lowered* "dangerous" triglycerides by 13 percent while, the low-fat diet *raised* them by 11 percent. Overall, the 35 percent-fat version lowered heart disease risk by 21 percent; the 20 percent diet only lowered the risk by 12 percent.

In another study, this one by researchers at the University of Rochester in New York, it was found that peanut butter and peanut oil were just as effective as olive oil (which has reigned as king of the healthful fats for years) in lowering blood levels of LDL cholesterol and triglycerides.

Maybe fat isn't the problem. Maybe, just maybe, fat is not the evil monster it has been portrayed to be. After all, fat is a necessary part of our diet and our body, too. There is only a problem with fat when we have or imbibe too much of it (or too little — fat chance of that) or the wrong kind. What is so good about fat? I'll tell you.

1. Our brain cells must be myelinated (sheathed in a *fatty* substance) in order to function efficiently.
2. Fat is our body's main source of energy.
3. Fat supports our internal organs and acts as a shock absorber to protect them.
4. Prostaglandins made from fat are required for calcium to enter bone cells. With insufficient dietary fat, stress fractures or osteoporosis may result.
5. Vitamins A, D, E and K are fat-soluble and rely on fat for absorption and utilization.
6. The various hormones, such as the human-growth hormone, testosterone and insulin, which regulate the body's processes and keep us youthful, are fat dependent.
7. The adipose tissue layer just under the skin is an insulator against extreme temperature changes and it also regulates the amount of moisture allowed into and out of the skin. Without this layer of fat, water soluble substances, such as chemical pollutants, would be able to more easily enter the body through the epidermis.
8. The body uses fat as a source of energy for heart muscle function. These fats, cholesterols and phospholipids, normally present in the heart muscle, generate energy to make the heart work more efficiently.
9. Finally, we just plain look better with a good, healthy ratio of fat to muscle.

We can't say that fat (with all its virtues) is our enemy just because some people ingest too much of it and/or die from heart attacks, any more than we can label water bad stuff just because countless people have drowned in it. In other words, it's not fat's fault that we get plump or sick any more than it is water's fault that we get wet.

Twenty or so years ago, health authorities looked at the large amount of fat that we were consuming and the fact that we as a people were getting fatter, and concluded that it was obvious that the one was causing the other. But they were wrong! They also looked at cholesterol and its connection to saturated fat. They studied our arteries and found dangerous triglycerides (fat) and cholesterol-laden plaque clogging our blood vessels and causing cardiovacular disease and heart attacks. Again they put two and two together and got four. Wrong again! They really only had three. Let me explain from my layman's point of view.

What we consume affects our hormonal balance. The endocrine system is an intricate network of ductless glands that produce a wide variety of hormones, with diverse and interrelated purposes. An increase or decrease in one hormone affects the others in a synergistic dance or interplay. For example, when cortisol (the "stress hormone") increases, the human-growth hormone and testosterone recede; when insulin spikes, glucagon becomes temporarily dormant.

Some foods are high glycemic, which means they cause blood-sugar levels to rise quickly and as a result, insulin to be released in relatively-large amounts. Other foods are medium or low glycemic and as such, result in a much smaller rise in blood sugar and a smaller insulin response/release. Dietary fat causes glucagon (insulin's antagonist/alter ego) to be released into the blood stream, supplanting the insulin, to burn fat for energy.

The body seeks stabilized blood-sugar levels because too high or low quantities of glucose in the blood is a danger to the survival of the organism. Thus, when we snack on a donut and a sugary soda, the sudden spike in our sugar level signals the body to go into emergency mode, releasing a relatively-large quantity of insulin to lower the amount of blood glucose. Since the high-sugar level is going to put the body into a sugar-burning mode (insulin release), any fat in the donut (now in our blood) will not be needed for energy and therefore will stay in the blood stream as triglycerides and cholesterol until it can be stored as fat. The overreaction by the insulin causes the blood sugar to be burned so thoroughly that the result is low blood sugar an hour or two later. This, likewise, is a dangerous situation, since the brain depends on glucose as its only source of energy. To get the sugar levels up again, the body/brain sends out hunger sensations or signals. As a result, more food and drink is craved and eaten. If the food/drink is mostly high glycemic again (as in a candy bar, soda, etc.) or a large meal, then the insulin response is another overreaction and the above scenario repeats itself. If we repeatedly eat a sugary/high-glycemic diet, eventually our insulin sensitivity is compromised and our blood lipids and cholesterol levels remain high, resulting in some of the surplus being deposited on/in the walls of the arteries as plaque; this is especially true if there are few antioxidants in the food and drink to prevent oxidation, that is, free radical damage that aids in the formation of risky cardiovascular plaques.

Another player in this drama is trans-fatty acids (alias hydrogenated fats, alias partially-hydrogenated oils). Trans-fats are very suspect. They are a creation of twentieth-century man — developed in the laboratory primarily to extend the shelf-life of vegetable oils and polyunsaturated fat and to give solidity to liquid oils. Butter is naturally-saturated fat; trans-fat is artificially, partially saturated by adding hydrogen atoms to its natural or original structure. Trans fats have been shown to raise cholesterol levels, lower HDL (the good guy), and raise LDL (the bad guy). They also interfere with the metabolism of essential fatty acids and the creation of "good" eicosanoids (hormone-like substances that help the immune response, blood clotting, inflammation, ...). The result of trans-fat research and development is stick and other solid margerines. Besides margarines, it can be found in many prepackaged foods, such as bread, crackers and cookies.

Saturated fat is the other supposed bad guy of fats. With few exceptions, it is found in animal-derived foods: meats, eggs, and dairy products. The fact that, the Eskimoes, the French, the Cretans, and our forefathers have fared well with a heavy dose of saturated fat means it is probably a bit player who relies on those around it on the stage of life to determine if it is a "good" or "bad" guy. For example, those individuals and societies with labor-intensive lives (read that exercise-saturated) tend to be able to get away with eating higher doses of saturated fats with minimal ill effects.

A hero among fats is Omega-3 fat. Omega-3 fats are thought to play a part in reducing mortality from cardiovascular disease in many populations around the world. Some studies have found it to be capable of lowering triglyceride (fat) levels in the blood. It may also have a blood-thinning (anticoagulant) effect, as well as improving insulin sensitivity (making it a potential weight-loss aid). Omega-3's can be found in fatty (cold-water) fish, such as salmon, trout, herring and sardines; it is also available from soy products, flaxseed, green-leafy vegetables, and nuts.

The bottom line is that fat by itself does not cause us to get fat or sick. Rather, when trans-fats, saturated fats, large meals, AND high-glycemic foods are teamed with a lack of exercise — THEN the problems begin.

The answer is to eat fat in moderation as our fitness champions do. Fill up with fruits, vegetables and whole grains; then add your protein sources: meats, fish, soy products, eggs, dairy (mostly low-fat versions), nuts and seeds. Finally, keep sweets, refined white flour products, refined sugar products, prepackaged foods, fast foods, junk foods, and soda pop to a minimum (this will almost automatically keep trans-fats and their potential dangers at a minimum — especially if we use butter judiciously, instead of margarines). Oh yes, use olive oil and canola oil when in need of vegetable oils for meals and recipes.

The above is basically what Warren, Carl, and June do and it seems to work for them.

Second-Hand Smoke And First-Hand Alcohol

Some of our Masters of Fitness used to smoke, but all of them quit before they became (and in order to become) a champion. Others had drinking problems, but they traded them in for an addiction to exercising, racing and feeling good. We all know that drinking in moderation or abstaining altogether are the best routes to take for our well-being. We also all know about smoking's dark side, even if some 50-some-year-old can claim ignorance of its negative-health consequences and get a jury of supposedly-sane folk to agree with him. Not just side with him, but agree with him to the tune of a 3 billion (that's billion with a "**b**") dollar settlement (but I digress). I'm not going to waste your time and mine on rehashing the downside (or any upside for that matter). It's enough to say that our Master Champs don't abuse alcohol or tobacco — period.

Is One Fluid As Good As The Next?

We know we need to drink plenty of fluids to maintain our well-being, but does it matter what we drink? We have access to teas, coffee, sodas, fruit juices, alcoholic beverages, hot chocolate and oh, yes, plain old water. Are any or all of these beverages, as effective as water for hydrating our systems? The experts say no. They say that nothing beats 100% pure water for quenching our thirst and meeting our body's needs. Some of our fitness champs (James and Helen come to mind) drink a lot of tea with their water and it just so happens that tea (green and basic black) has gotten some good press lately concerning human longevity and its being a good source of antioxidants.

Caffeinated beverages, whether they be coffee, cola, or ..., and alcoholic drinks dehydrate the body, acting as diuretics and leading to fatigue, indigestion, muscle cramps and headaches. Many nutritionists recommend that we drink an extra glass of water for each caffeinated or alcoholic beverage we imbibe; that's in addition to the recommended 8-to-10 glasses per day. That's what the "experts" tell us. What do our Masters of Fitness do? Although *they don't normally drink sodas*, some of them do down them during marathons and ultras for the energy boost they get from the caffein and/or sugar. Also, Ruth Anderson and running's guru, George Sheehan, would enjoy a beer together after marathon runs as an enjoyable "recovery drink." Why beer? Maybe because in moderation: * It resupplies the B vitamins lost due to the stress of a long run * Replenishes fluids and "calories" * The alcohol "magnifies" the sense of accomplishment and good feelings associated with one's successful effort.

Some experts go as far as to claim that carbonated beverages/soda pop interfere with digestion and weaken our bones. A study at Boston's Children's Hospital found that an extra soft drink each day increases a child's chances of becoming obese by 60 percent. Our question is: Does this "liquid sugar" have a similar effect on those of us who are a little older?

Ed Mayhew with Mary Mayhew

When we drink beverages other than water, the body has to use some of the water contained in that drink to counteract the impurities, toxins, ... (such as, caffeine, alcohol, phosphoric acid, refined sugar, artificial coloring) that the drink is delivering. On the other hand, 100 percent of a glass of pure water can be utilized for delivery to the cells for use in their metabolic processes.

Water is the main transporter of nutrients to the trillions of cells in the body. It also carries wastes from the cells and out of the body in the sweat, expiration and urine. Other functions include maintaining the body's optimal temperature, lubricating joints, and keeping lungs moist for more efficient breathing. Water regulates histamine to prevent or alleviate allergies, asthma and chronic pain. Slight dehydration can slow our metabolism by three percent and cause mental confusion. According to a report by the Health Care Financing Administration, dehydration is a major cause of hospitalization in people over 65.

Our fitness champions drink a variety of fluids (including water) in moderate-to-heavy amounts. James stays well hydrated drinking 32 ounces of orange juice at breakfast; 32 oz. of water or unsweetened tea for lunch; 32 oz. of water or unsweetened tea with dinner; 20 oz. of Gatorade in the afternoon; AND 16 oz. more of water throughout the day. During races (on warm days in particular) he loads up on 16 oz. of water just before the race (on top of his breakfast o.j.) and tries to down 8 oz. per mile during his marathons. That's a lot of fluid — I wonder if James holds any Johnny Blue stock?

Norm, on the other hand, took fluids much more sparingly. Norm only took fluids at the marathon distance (none on shorter runs/races) and just at the hydration stops through miles 15 or 18. During training he ran without fluids as part of his "no water during a race" discipline. Normally, Norm consumes 10 to 12 ounces at each of three meals in a day with possibly a similar quantity once or twice at other times. Now he realizes that he was chronically dehydrated during his racing career, but that's the way he trained and his stash of medals, trophies and world records are testaments to the success of his approach.

You can see that there is a wide disparity from one champion to the next, but they all drank and drink at least moderate amounts of health-promoting beverages. Those competing in ultras drank (and ate) "constantly" during their races (including sodas) in order to keep on keeping on. None of them make a habit of drinking sodas on a regular basis, except possibly during a *long* race or training run. Several drink teas, coffees and fruit juices (frequently, but not during ultras) AND *all* drink substantial amounts of pure water, all of the time.

Food Supplements

You probably know someone who frequents the local health food stores taking this vitamin and that latest miracle potion; yet, they never seem to get any better, fitter or healthier. You may also be acquainted with some robust, healthy individuals who swear by their supplement regimen. Do supplements help or don't they? Are they really necessary for optimal fitness and good health? Let's look to our fitness champions for answers.

James rid himself of several extra pounds and dangerously-high blood pressure by turning himself into an outstanding runner and champion marathoner without taking any vitamins, herbs, or pharmaceutical aids at all. Last year, after 6 years of successful racing, he started taking a multi-vitamin for health insurance, just in case he wasn't getting all his nutrients.

Helen, over a 23-year span, ran about 200 races of marathon distance or longer (much longer) while staying completely injury free. During this time she took no food supplements (as in "none"). Since then, she's started taking antioxidants at the prompting of the aerobics "czar," Dr. Kenneth Cooper. Although her heart, lungs and bones were found to be those of a 30-year-old, her skin had taken a beating over the years of running in the sun, wind and rain/snow/sleet/hail/you-name-it. Thus, the recommendation to begin supplementing at age 75.

Jerry ran his 200-marathon marathon with the aid of just two supplements. One was Barley Essence, which in *essence* is just a convenient way (powder added to water) to take top-quality, health-and energy-promoting greens. The other, Endurox R4, is an electrolyte and energy-replenishing drink somewhat similar to Gatorade. He has since added glucosamine/chondroitin because of stiffness in his knees (gee, I wonder why he got that?)

Warren and Ruth have taken vitamin E for years as nutritional insurance. Other of our champions take a small variety of different food supplements. There's not one "potion" or type of nutritional supplement that all or even several of them take that we can point to and say, "so that's their secret!" My thinking is that if these individuals who are just like us, only fitter, can accomplish what they have without taking handfuls of "vitamins," then maybe we can too. If our diet is as excellent as theirs, then maybe we too can excel with a minimum of supplementation.

Remember, if we start taking a particular nutrient in pill form, over time the body may become lazy and start depending on it. Eventually it may lose its ability to manufacture this nutrient from other raw materials obtained from the foods we eat.

A good multi-vitamin/mineral supplement, which June recommends, is good health insurance and might be worth the investment, but an unending array of vitamins and herbs might just empty your pockets. Of course, if we have a condition that can be helped by supplementation (or, if you are a bodybuilder), then that might be a course worth pursuing. However, our master fitness champs have shown us that their high level of fitness and their awe-inspiring accomplishements in the athletic arena came from a quality diet, not a pill bottle.

Eat What You Like — Like What You Eat

Broccoli may be chockful of beneficial nutrients, but if we can't stomach it, then why eat it? Life is too short to have to endure self-inflicted misery. Not only that, but we don't stick with a food that we can't stand unless we're a little masochistic; and the most nutritious food in the world won't do us much good unless we consume it on a regular basis. We can't very well say, "I ate a helping of carrots last groundhogs' day, so I have my vitamin A for this lifetime."

There is a huge variety of fruits, vegetables, whole grains, protein sources, etc. available to us. Find ones that you like and partake of them often. Enjoying what we eat actually makes us fitter. Remember, when we don't enjoy what we are dining on, that negative feeling is telling us that we are in a catabolic state (a breaking down of the body), or heading there. Likewise, when we are savoring our meal, that positive experience or emotion is a sign that we are in or approaching, an anabolic state (a building up of the body, including musculature and mental acumen). Just as bad as eating something that makes us borderline nauseated is devouring something we know is not good for us. The feelings of guilt or remorse tell us we have set sail for Catabolic Island.

As we've said, depriving ourselves of what we like to eat never works for long. That is why it is a good idea to have one day a week when we can eat that cheesecake or juicy, triple bacon, cheeseburger deluxe. Knowing that we ate well all week allows us to enjoy that once-a-week treat, that Hot Fudge Brownie Supreme, without the guilt we feel when we "cheat" on a regular basis. Plan ahead; plan a week of nutritious, bodybuilding, health-building meals, but don't forget that special treat day. Telling ourselves that we will never again feast on a favorite, decadent dessert is a recipe for failure. Knowing we can occasionally eat our favorite unhealthful snacks helps keep us on the path to a fitter self the rest of the time. Also, these once-a-week splurges help remind us of how uncomfortably full, bloated and gross we feel when we overeat or make poor eating choices. These weekly binges help us appreciate our daily healthful culinary fare, by reminding us of how much better we feel when we eat well. None of the fitness champions that I interviewed appears to be a "purist" when it comes to diet; they all have their occasional treat and more — as should we.

CHAPTER 7 THE 60-SECOND SOLUTION

I know what you are thinking, "What can be accomplished in just 60 seconds? This is ridiculous! First, the fitness experts and exercise-equipment-and-program promoters (otherwise known as the snake-oil salesmen of the second half of the twentieth century) told us that we needed 45 minutes to an hour per session to get in shape; then they sold us on 30-minutes a day; next came 20 minutes, followed closely by 15 minutes to rock-hard abs, buns, etc.; 10 minutes at a time was the mantra of the experts recently; finally, at the checkout counter in a supermarket today an 8-minute program was being endorsed. Now you have the audacity to suggest a 60-second workout. What can we possibly accomplish in one minute, Mayhew?"

First, I am not promoting 60-second exercise sessions as the ultimate in body-building. Second, exercise is not center stage in this chapter; instead we are talking about how we can finally stop procrastinating when it comes to exercise and just as important, what we can do to see that we stick with a workout program until we can get the results we desire and deserve. This is where most of us drop the exercise-ball. We all know that we should be exercising on a regular basis, but a little thing called life seems to keep getting in the way. Our focus with the 60-Second Solutions is to find out what we can do to *finally get started* and *persevere* with a program so that we can reap the life-changing benefits year after year after year.

What can we accomplish in just 60 seconds? In a mere 60 seconds or less we can bless our food, say a prayer, recite a poem, or pledge allegiance to the flag. We can give or receive a heartfelt compliment; write a quick thank-you note. We can smile, say hi, and greet several people we meet at the store or at the office AND as a result, brighten their day just a little. We can tell a teacher, coach or mentor how much of a difference their work and caring has made in a child's life. On the flip side, we can make a nasty or biting, sarcastic remark that will never, ever be forgotten. We can complain, moan and groan about our lot in life or some petty grievance.

What else can we do in just 60-seconds of time?

1. In 60 seconds we can imagine mowing the grass and decide that that's good enough for today.
2. In 60 seconds *or less* we can walk from one room to another to get something and when we get there forget what we are there for.
3. We can bend down at the store to check out a canned good on the bottom shelf and realize that we may need the assistance of a forklift to get back up.
4. In a scant 60 seconds we can whip out our plastic and painlessly purchase a $1,000 thingamajig that we'll be paying for months later when said doohickey is collecting dust in the attic.
5. Travel a mile in our car only to realize that we left our husband in the service-station restroom.

Life is just one moment after another. Said another way, it is merely one 60-second segment after another until we've filled yet another day. We can waste these brief, precious segments of time (and thus the days of our lives) or we can make them count.

60-Second Freeze-Framing

The Institute of HeartMath has done some remarkable research, much of which has been published in prestigious, peer-reviewed professional journals. You can read about their research and programs in chapter 8. Their founder, Doc Lew Childre, created a *one-minute stress-reduction technique* called Freeze-Framing that can change one's heart rate variability (HRV) from an incoherent (stressed state) to a coherent pattern (stress-free state).

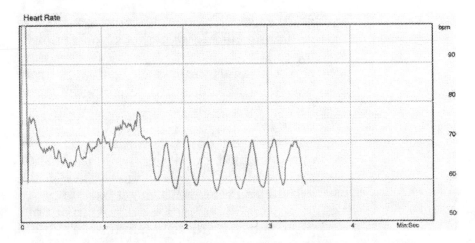

Author's HRV from incoherent (anger state) to a coherent, stress-free pattern in just seconds using a 60-Second Solution — Freeze-Frame

An incoherent HRV signal sends a message from the heart to the body and brain that there is a life-threatening situation. After all, the heart is the focal point of our well-being and it is not running smoothly or pumping efficiently. The individual is heading towards or is already in a pro-aging catabolic state; the body is preparing for "fight or flight" in order to survive. In contrast, when the heart is producing a coherent HRV, this signals the brain and body that all is well and therefore it is a good time for the body to use its energies and reserves to build and repair tissues and cells; this is the anti-aging, anabolic state we desire.

In its research, using "mental" techniques such as this, the Institute of HeartMath has been able to show an average increase of 100 percent in DHEA (the "fountain of youth" hormone) and an average cortisol (the "stress" hormone) decrease of 23 percent in test subjects in about a month's time. In another study at the IHM, participants who focused for just 5 minutes on something they appreciated had their IgA (Immunoglobulin A — part of the immune system's first line of defense) elevated for several hours. In contrast, those who were instructed to focus on a stressor experienced a depression of their IgA for a similar length of time.

174

Yes, we can accomplish much in a mere 60 seconds (or 5 consecutive 60-second segments, as above). Whether we use our minute(s): to give a heartfelt thank you or to complain; to pray or to bemoan our predicament; to Freeze-Frame or to get a stress-induced headache; to appreciate our loved ones or to leave our mate behind in a service station lavatory — we can be assured that what we do with our minutes will make a significant difference in our life!

60-Second Solution #1 — Counting Our Blessings

When we truly appreciate something, we tend to take care of it whether it be a car, an outfit *or ourselves*. The object of this 60-second Solution is to count our blessings or acknowledge what we appreciate so that we can attract more of it. For example, kids who like baseball or other trading cards end up getting more and more of them because, like us, what they focus upon grows. Likewise, have you noticed that women who like shoes have closets full of them, whereas men who don't give a hoot about their footwear will wear the same 2 or 3 pair day after day? Have you ever noticed that when you start complaining about something, more things to moan and bitch about pop into your mind? In a like manner, with our loving thoughts come more and more loving thoughts. Similarly, thoughts and feelings of appreciation will bring us more of the well-being that we desire.

It is easier, at first, (but not essential) to do these 60-Second Solutions with the eyes closed to shut out distractions that might detour our thinking. Take a deep, relaxing breath and let it out slowly, savoring its deliciousness. Repeat two or three times. Now think, "one" and see the number one in your mind's eye. Now think about something that you appreciate (e.g., your home). *Feel* your appreciation for this item or subject. This is most important, feeling the good feeling associated with this thought. Next, silently say, "two" and think of something else you appreciate. Only this time, it has to be an aspect of yourself. It could be your eyes: their appearance or the quality of your vision. Remember, getting in touch with the positive feelings is the key. Continue this process to ten, making every even-numbered item something you like about yourself. The harder it is for you to think of that which you appreciate about yourself, the more you will benefit from this 60-Second Solution. As your appreciation for yourself grows, you will find yourself wanting to take better care of yourself. You will naturally want to eat better and exercise more.

Count Your Blessings before each meal or snack; when you first get in your car or at stoplights (eyes wide open); right before bed or as you wake up. Have set daily events or times that trigger your 60-SS.

If you happen to be one of those myriad of individuals who think, "there is nothing to appreciate about my body; I have so many ailments; I'm so fat, etc." — think again. Remember, if your body/mind were not doing many more things "right than wrong," you would be a former inhabitant of the planet Earth. Right now your immune system is successfully battling countless harmful microorganisms and your trillions of cells are dutifully carrying out their functions on your behalf.

Will this simplistic little technique work? How can merely thinking about things make a difference? Don't I need to *do* something? You are doing something when you take 60 seconds here and there throughout your day to get into a feeling of appreciation. A study at Yale University supports this thinking when it found that depressed patients felt much better when they merely *imagined* someone they respected praising them.

Remember, the mind does not differentiate between that which is vividly imagined and that which is actually experienced in the concrete world. An experiment at Manchester Metropolitan University in England by sports psychologist Dave Smith, Ph.D. proved this once again. He compared three groups: one that exercised; another that didn't; and a third that only *thought* about muscle contractions twenty times per day. The actual exercisers increased their strength by 33 percent, while those who didn't exercise at all had no improvement, as expected. Significantly, those who just did the exercises mentally had an astonishing 16 percent improvement in strength. Interestingly, Dr. Smith found that if the mental exercisers allowed their mind to wander at all, the technique didn't work.

According to Herbert Benson, M.D., associate professor of medicine at Harvard Medical School, remembered wellness is a powerful tool for restoring health. Brain researchers have found that just thinking about a physical activity produces the same pattern of activity in the brain as does actually performing the activity. The brain sends signals to the body that causes it to react the same to mental images as it does to actual physical events. We experience this when we go to the movies and afterwards find our muscles all tense and tired out as if we were the one doing battle with the bad guys on the screen.

Finally, to benefit from 60-Second Solution #1, from time to time during your day, take just 60 seconds to mentally *appreciate* 10 things — emphasizing and savoring the good feelings!

60-Second Solution #2 - Be A Why's Guy

If the why is strong enough, we will find a way. Find the most important reason why you want or need to be fit and focus on it for one full minute and you will amp up your desire. If it is so you can play tag with your grandchildren and great-grandchildren, see yourself doing it in your mind's eye. Use all your senses. Smell the fresh-mown grass. Feel the ground under your feet as you dart and dodge to avoid being tagged. See the smiles on your grandchildren's faces. Hear the laughter and the giggles of sheer delight. See the colors of their eyes, clothes and the blue sky. When you are done playing, hear them saying, "I love you, Grandpa/Grandma. You're the best grandma/grandpa in the whole wide world," as they hug you as only a small child can do. Most importantly, *feel* the joy and delight. Going to this 60-second mental-movie theater several times a day and imagining this or some other event as if it were actually happening for the sheer joy of the imaginings themselves *will do more to get you eating "right" and working out than just about anything else you could possibly do!*

Maybe you would rather fantasize about running your first marathon to raise money for a worthy cause. Imagine what it would be like to have family and friends cheering you on. Listen as they congratulate you; see them beaming with joy over your accomplishment as you cross the finish line. Think about the sense of pride and accomplishment. How does it feel to do something you and others thought was absolutely impossible just a few months previously? Use all your senses to mentally experience your first marathon, with the emphasis on how it feels. Focus on the positive feelings of accomplishment and support, not the obstacles, like the aching feet, etc. Again, go to this joyful place several times a day, 60 seconds or so at a time. As mentioned before, have set times to do this, such as during bathroom breaks, as well as spontaneous sessions. Enjoy!

60-Second Solution #3 - Consider It Done

When our belief and desire on a subject coalesce, our wish manifests. However, if we desire something to happen, but our belief that it can happen is weak, we feel negative emotions (perhaps frustration or futility) and we will often procrastinate because deep down we don't think (or believe) that our taking action would accomplish much. A less-powerful desire teamed with a lack of belief just produces mild frustration or irritation and again, little action. On the other hand, our belief can be strong while our desire is lacking; in this case, there is little initiative to take action. Nothing much happens in these scenarios and for good reason — our desire and belief on a topic are not in sync. In contrast, a powerful desire that teams up with a potent belief produces passion, excitement, unbridled enthusiasm, *and action* that produces the goods. Things just seem to fall into place; foul-ups and roadblocks are few and easily rectified. In this state we are in "the flow," or in what some call "the Zone."

You have the desire to be fitter after 50 or you wouldn't be reading this book. We can goose up that desire by performing 60-Second Solution #2 - Be A Why's Man. However, if you feel that your desire is already burning brightly, then your belief that you can get fitter than most 20-year-olds must be impotent or you would already be an awesome specimen/FA50.

Consider-It-Done is the 60-Second Solution that builds our belief that our efforts will indeed bear fruit; that our efforts at a significant transformation will not be in vain. It is the notion that nothing will really come of our efforts that keeps us from starting and/or persevering.

Imagine you are already as trim, muscular or energetic as you would like to be. Imagine that right now you are experiencing that awesome state of fitness. See yourself entering the foyer for your __th high school or college reunion. Look in the giant wall mirror, and see, in detail, how well your tux, gown or other outfit shows off your envy-producing, brand-new physique or figure. Hear the murmers and gasps, see the heads turn, accept the sincere compliments, and acknowledge the epidemic of jaw-dropping, eye-popping looks that you are getting. You've never looked better — ever! Notice your hair, the healthful glow of your skin, your radiance. Feel it all for the pure joy it gives you to do so. Of course, this is just one option. Maybe instead you are running along the beach, lounging under a beach umbrella, or strolling in the moonlight. Go back to the beach often in your imagination just for the sheer joy it brings you. Notice how good you look strolling down the beach in your bathing suit, a bounce in your step, a smile on your face, able to keep up with the grandchildren, enjoying life. Don't take this mental journey to make it actually happen. That just causes you to look in the mirror and see that it hasn't happened yet, wonder why it hasn't, get frustrated that it is not "real" yet, etc. Instead, enjoy the 60 seconds for the fun of enjoying the 60 seconds and know that when desire and belief align, things will start popping and it won't be the buttons popping off your clothiing due to girth expansion.

Actually, as you probably noticed, 60-Second Solutions #2 and #3 are virtually identical except for their purposes — to rev up desire or to strengthen belief. In Truth, they do both at the same time. How do we know if we are doing the "exercise" correctly? If we are *enjoying* the 60 seconds, we are successfully goosing up our desire and establishing the belief that we really can be fitter after 50!

Do Our Masters Of Fitness Do This?

Jerry Dunn, "America's Marathon Man" mentally sees a scene that is upcoming miles down the road before he actually gets there. This helps propel him to that forthcoming section of the marathon route. In essence, he's imaging what it would be like to be at mile 20 when he's at mile marker 16, for instance. This helps keep him moving forward when he's dragging a little.

Golfers, high jumpers, gymnasts and basketball free-throw shooters (the good ones) always go through their performance mentally right before they execute it physically on the field of play. We always accomplish our goals mentally before the physical manifestation.

Our Masters Of Fitness are successful in races from 100-meter sprints to 6-day ultras, at posing for bodybuilding competitions and in 100-mile mountain bike rides because they have the desire to succeed and the belief that they can. They *mentally* and physically prepare for each challenge they choose to undertake. If our own desires and beliefs were as synchronized (as one) as theirs are in the fitness and health arena, then we would be enjoying a similar level of achievement. They may not need these 60-Second Solutions because they do the same mental gymnastics naturally, almost automatically, in their everyday life. They are succeeding because of the way they see themselves and life. Unless our fitness is already on par with theirs, we can train ourselves to think more like they do by using these simple, yet powerful 60-SS techniques. The more we use them, at least several times a day, the more ready and eager we will be to do what needs to be done in the area of lifestyle enhancements (exercise, diet, attitudes, stress reduction, ...) to be fitter after 50.

Prayer — A 60-Second Solution

I mention prayer here because it can be a powerful 60-Second Solution to our desire for well-being for ourselves and others, when it is a heartfelt request imbued by faith. Faith being the belief and appreciation that all prayers are answered. "The substance of things hoped for, the evidence of things not yet seen" is a famous description of the faith that gives prayer its power.

Science is beginning to discover that prayer really does work. For example, Dr. Rogerio Lobo, chairman of obstetrics and Gynecology at Columbia University College of Physicians and Surgeons and his colleagues recently performed an experiment that showed the effectiveness of prayer. It involved 199 women in South Korea who were attempting to have a baby by use of in-vitro fertilization procedures and embyo transfers due to infertility problems. Unbeknownst to the women and their attending physicians, the scientists had arranged for a few individuals in the United States, Canada, and Australia to pray on behalf of some of the women, for a three-week period.

The unwitting subjects were divided into two groups; the individuals in the one group were prayed for and those in the other were not. The results were impressive: Those supported by prayer had a 50 percent pregnancy rate compared to only 26 percent for those not getting this assistance. This despite the fact that none of the women nor their doctors knew about the experiment. Making this study even more credible is the fact that it wasn't tainted by the set agenda of a pro-prayer organization. In other words, it wasn't conducted, requested, or funded by a religious group, but rather it was designed and controlled by those highly skeptical folks — scientists!

Music — 60 Seconds Or More
Music greatly affects our moods and as we have discussed, our emotions or moods let us know whether we are "aging" our body or rejuvenating it. According to noted health expert, Deepak Chopra, M.D., if we wish to lower our blood pressure, listening to slow, classical music will do so. Dr. Chopra also tells of attending a medical conference where another doctor was able, at will, to raise and lower the pulse rates of all the attending physicians simply by singing different songs.

Research at the Institute of HeartMath has shown that properly-designed music can increase DHEA, reduce cortisol and improve the balance and coherence of the autonomic nervous system (ANS). The ANS can regulate every aspect of the immune system by regulating the production of the body's immuno-modulatory hormones. See chapter 8 for more information on IHM research and programs.

Music, whether sung, played, conducted, listened to, danced to or exercised to can put us in a youthfulness-inducing anabolic state or minimize and/or shorten a catabolic (aging) state. However, when it comes to music, often one person's joy is another person's misery. Music that would inspire a teenager may drive a 60-year-old to distraction or worse. Some music is more universally beneficial, such as certain classical baroque pieces or the specially-designed music produced by the Institute of HeartMath, but it really is a matter of individual choice. Choose music that invigorates or relaxes you, depending on the circumstances. The right music gets you moving, working out at your most productive level. Use it to get up and out of your easy chair, and out the door or to make your exercise sessions more fun, because if your exercise sessions are fun, you will be more likely to stay motivated and to stick with them. And, it only takes *a minute* or two to select and pop in a cassette or CD that will make all the difference.

If feasible, throughout the day, play your favorite tunes to enhance the effectiveness of your 60-Second Solution sessions. If the music is a distraction, then that is a sign to go with silence.

Laughter — A 60-Second Solution

Research at the University of Maryland Medical Center in Baltimore found that those who had suffered a heart attack or had bypass surgery were 40 percent less likely to laugh than were individuals in good cardiovascular health. Even when things were going well the heart patients were less likely to laugh and more likely to become angry.

Earlier studies have proven that a good sense of humor can strengthen the immune system and lessen inflammation of the heart. Laughter increases the concentration of circulating antibodies and white blood cells for fighting foreign proteins that have invaded the body.

A study at the Loma Linda University School of Medicine found that test subjects who watched a humorous 60-minute video had significant reductions in their stress hormones — cortisol and adrenaline. These hormones in excess can exacerbate a host of stress-related maladies, such as depression and heart disease.

Other controlled studies at Loma Linda by Lee Berk and Stanley Tan showed that laughter also increases T lymphocytes, the number and activity level of natural killer cells, and the number of T cells that have helper/suppresser receptors. What this all means in layman's terms is a greatly strengthened immune system that can attack and annihilate renegade viral and cancer cells (among others) that are always lurking in the body and looking to gain a foothold.

Other studies have shown that humor and laughter can block pain by unleashing a flood of endorphins — one of the body's natural pain killers. One such experiment was conducted at Bar-Ilan University in Israel; two-hundred subjects were shown one of three videos (one funny, the others not). A half hour later the group that had watched the comedy were able to submerge their hands in ice water for 51 seconds — 17 seconds longer than the other two video groups and 11 seconds longer than a fourth group that saw no video at all.

Salivary immunoglobulin A is a first line of defense against invading microorganisms. Research at Western New England College found that subjects had increased concentrations of IgA after viewing funny videos. In a related study at the University of Waterloo, Onterio, participants who scored well on a test for appreciation and the utilization of humor had even higher levels of IgA after watching a funny video.

According to humor researcher Dr. William Fry, all the major systems of the body, including the respiratory, cardiovascular, muscular, endocrine, and the immune system, are benefitted by mirthful laughter.

Years ago, Type A individuals (e.g., the hard-driving executive) were thought to be prone to heart disease and heart attacks, but subsequent studies have shown that only *angry* Type A's are at risk. Further proving this finding is a six-year study of 13,000 adults reported in the Spring of 2000 in *Circulation*, a journal of the American Heart Association. It revealed that those most prone to anger were 2.69 times more likely to have a heart attack or die of heart disease. Needless to say (but I'll say it anyway) people who learn to laugh at themselves and diffuse situations by finding the humor in them are not likely to become hotheads or depressed. The message is simple — learn to laugh at life. Make sure your day is filled with chuckles, guffaws, belly laughs, giggles, smiles, and winks.

One 60-Second Solution is to get a 365-day calender that has a different joke or cartoon on each day's page and take 60 seconds or so to enjoy the joke of the day. Make it a habit to laugh at those E-mailed or internet jokes that abound (But don't do it on company time because losing your job would be *no-laughing* matter). If you like Jay Leno or David Letterman but don't want to stay up that late, tape the monologue and watch it the next day. Crank up the VCR and tape some reruns of the classics: The Andy Griffith Show, I Love Lucy, Bill Cosby,

Dean Martin and Jerry Lewis, or ... to watch when you need or want a laugh or two. Get your hands on some old radio classic cassettes of the Jack Benny Show or Fibber Magee and Molly and listen to them while driving in the car. Keep some funny books and/or magazines handy for an impromptu chortle or two (and what could be better than a good rib-tickling chortle?). In other words, enjoy some good belly laughs every day for a fitter you.

Reward Yourself

A near-foolproof way to insure our sticking with our fitness plans is to set goals and subgoals and reward ourselves when we reach them. Who else will? Yes, the race directors will when we get good enough to place, and that trophy or medal will mean a lot and motivate us more than we think. It is not the medal itself, but what it stands for that will drive us. Until then, here is a program to keep us on track to the fitness we've always wanted.

First, decide on some prizes that you would like to receive, that you can afford to give yourself AND that you can and will wait for until you have earned them. For example, let's say for argument's sake that there is a piece of clothing you want. You purchase it and put it where you can see it; but you don't get to wear it until you've reached the fitness goal that you have set for yourself (the dangling carrot rouse). Or you don't even get to purchase the reward until you have reached your goal.

Make a list of all the possible rewards that interest you: tickets to the movies/theater, a meal at a special restaurant, a trip, something special for the car (preferably not something the car won't run without), a pedicure, a massage, jewelry, a book, shoes, or even a trophy (engraved of course) or certificate that you design on your computer or order specially made. Some prizes should be commensurate with sub-goals and some with major goals.

Now that you have your prizes picked out, set some goals and sub-goals for your fitness quest. It's best not to have a goal of exercisng for a set number of *consecutive* days, for example, because if you miss a single day, you are back to square one and usually demoralized by your *failure*. Instead, set goals that deal with totals (e.g., when I have exercised a total of thirty days, I will reward myself with a new outfit); that

184

way, even if you miss five days of exercise, you could still reach your goal, only now it would take thirty-five days' time (i.e., thirty exercise days plus five non-exercise days). This way you never have to start over because of a lapse or two.

Have subgoals that lead up to your major goal. If the big-goal is to start eating six fruits and vegetables every day and to make this a major lifestyle change and a lifelong habit, then break this goal into smaller, easily-achieved segments. For example, you've decided that this goal will have been achieved when you have eaten six or more fruits and veggies on 40 of the next 43 days. Your smaller segment or subgoal is five days of consuming six f & v. Each time you reach this mini-goal you will reward yourself by having one piece of your favorite dessert or by buying some trinket. These smaller, more frequent rewards help us to stay motivated until we can reach our big goal and its major intrinsic and extrinsic rewards.

Make this goal/commitment in writing. Place it where you can read it and recommit daily. Use a calendar or chart to keep track of your progress and keep it in a prominent place. Remember, your goals need to be measurable. That means they involve numbers. With numbers we can see our progress and be inspired to follow through or see our lack of movement and know to make some adjustments.

Some would say that only intrinsic rewards are good; that the fitness goal itself is enough. But, tell me, if you didn't get paid for your job or your business continued to lose money, how long would you continue to report to work each Monday? Getting paid for what we do is an extrinsic reward that drives us to persist in our job through some tough times, doesn't it? If Helen Klein hadn't received a trophy, a T-shirt, and her picture in the paper at the end of her first 10-miler, would she have gone on to national prominence? I rest my case!

Now decide how you will reward yourself if (no, make that "when") you have followed through with your workout plan or diet guidelines.

Write it out: "I, _____, on my word of honor, pledge to exercise _____, and when I do, I promise to reward myself with a _____." Sign and date this document. By putting your commitment in writing, you have made a binding contract with yourself. Now if your word is worth anything, you are bound to follow through.

That's Interesting

When someone says something that irks us, instead of thinking, "You idiot!" or worse, we can think to ourself, "that's interesting" or "isn't that interesting" or "that *is really* interesting!" By just *observing* their contrasting political, moral, or religious viewpoint rather than getting irritated and pushing against it, we can maintain an internal chemical balance that supports our well-being. When we verbally or even mentally (our expressions and body language give us away) do battle with them, we strengthen their resolve (people automatically push back, mentally or physically, when "pushed") and weaken our connection with our Source Energy, our well-being/fitness. Our desires are born out of the contrast and diverse points of view. Vive La Difference!

Calendar

At the start of each week, record your appointments to exercise like you record all your other important engagements. Treat them as you would a meeting with your boss, a business lunch with a client, or your kid's soccer game. Decide that there has to be a major conflict before you will even think about cancelling a scheduled workout. Record other items important to your fitness/health, such as dietary commitments, rest and relaxation appointments, massages, and the like. Also note your fitness accomplishments on the calendar. For example, record how many minutes you actually biked on Thursday and compare it with your original plan. This calendar technique helps keep us consistent in our exercising, eating well, etc. and consistency is the name of the game. Without the calendar we can easily wake up one day to find that we haven't exercised for two or three weeks.

The 60-Second Workout Solution

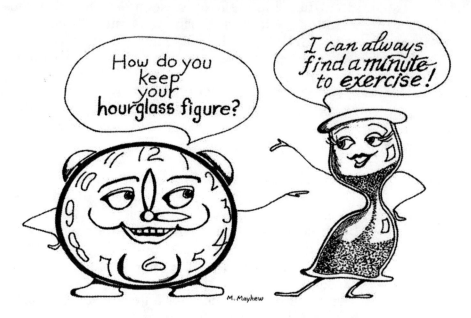

As I said before, I am not suggesting that 60-second snippets of exercise is the best way to go. Ten, twenty and forty-five-minute workouts are definitely better, but to make it easy for you to get started, here are a few 60-second exercises that can be done almost anytime — anywhere for maximum convenience and to take away all time-related excuses for not exercising. Once you've gotten moving, you can switch to a more substantial program, such as those in the next chapter.

First, here is a reminder of the importance of even a little physical movement for our well-being. The Japanese government recently did a study of what is being called "economy-class syndrome." This is where airline passengers develop deep-vein thrombosis or the formation of blood clots due to their lack of muscular movement during long, cramped flights. The report says, in essence, that 100 to 150 passengers arriving at Tokyo's Narita Airport suffer from this condition each year, and that in the previous eight years 25 passengers had actually died from ECS. A few 60-second exercise sessions may have been able to prevent these health problems and deaths.

Just what can a mere 60 seconds of exercise accomplish? Well, weightlifters/bodybuilders only spend a handful of minutes in strenuous exertion during a typical hour-long session of weight training. They usually do a particular exercise, such as the bench press, for just 20 to 30 seconds (with only a handful of these seconds at maximum effort). Then they rest for a minute or two before doing another set. This new set is often working a different part of the body. From this, we can see that working a specific set of muscles for a mere 60 seconds can get results.

The 60-Second Exercise Solution Guidelines
1. These 60-SS exercises may be brief, but they are potent bodybuilders for anyone who has been fairly sedentary for a while. Therefore, only do these barbell-free strength builders every other day; alternate them with aerobic workouts (walks, runs, ...) on the other days.
2. Two or three repetitions of an exercise with each arm or leg is more than enough.
3. Silently and slowly count to seven while contracting the muscle (bending the arms or legs, for example); and then count to seven while extending or straightening the arm or leg and returning it to the starting position.
4. Keep breathing throughout the exercise. Do NOT hold your breath. Holding your breath can put an unnecessary stress and strain on the bodily systems and raise the blood pressure.
5. The resistance in these strength-building exercises comes from one arm or leg resisting the other one. Apply as much resistance as you can so as to make the muscles work very hard for maximum results.
6. It is not necessary to do all these exercises each strength-training day. Just make sure that by the end of the week you've worked your upper and lower legs, pushing and pulling muscles of the arms, the back, and the abs.

7. Put on music when time and circumstances permit. Focus on the exercise itself and your body's effort.

8. When doing the stretches, hold each one for about 20 to 30 seconds; to avoid injury, never bounce or jerk the muscles. Always perform gentle movements (such as walking) to warm the muscles before stretching them. Relax into each stretch, keep breathing, and *enjoy* the gentle stretch — the limbering feeling.

Strength — The 60-Second Solution

Exercises we can do with little or no time, equipment, space, or gym memberships.

1. The Bench-less Press (pushing — strengthens arms and chest)

Start with the right arm bent and the right hand close to and in front of the right shoulder with the palm facing forward and fingers up. Make a fist with the left hand and place it in the palm of the right hand, with the left hand's palm facing down.

Straighten the right arm while the left resists and tries to prevent the right from straightening. Push as hard as you can with your right arm while resisting close to maximally with the left. Take about 7 seconds (a slow, silent count to 7) to fully straighten the right arm. Then immediately reverse the process so that the left arm is now trying to return the right to the starting position while the right arm resists (a 7-second return).

Repeat this press with the right arm 1 or 2 more times and then 2 or 3 times with the left arm pressing, making sure to breathe throughout this whole exercise and all the exercises that follow: exhale on the first 7-second press; and inhale as the arm returns to its starting position.

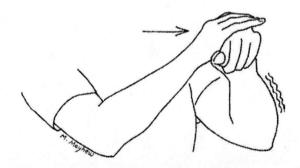

near hand pushes and
far hand resists until arms
are straight

2. The Machine-less Row (pulling — strengthens arms and back)

Stretch the arms straight out in front of the chest. With the palms facing down, grab the left wrist/hand with the right hand and, left hand resisting, start pulling the the left hand to the right side of the chest (about nipple high) until the left hand's thumb touches right <u>side</u> of chest (both hands are to the right of right nipple). Then return the left hand to the starting position while the right arm tries to keep it at chest or hold it back. Do this exercise 2 or 3 times with the right arm and then 2 or 3 times with the left. *See 60-Second Exercise Solution Guidelines.

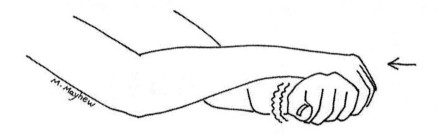

top hand pulls
while bottom hand resists
until hands are close to
shoulder

3. **Dumbbell-free Curls** (curling — strengthens biceps/upper arms)

Hang the right arm down so that the right hand's pinkie touches the outside of the right leg. With the palm of the right hand facing forward and fingers pointing down, put the fingers of the left hand in the palm of the right (for comfort and maximum strengthening of the arm, put a grapefruit or orange in the right hand for the left to grasp and push against) to resist the curling/bending of the right arm. Keeping the right elbow against the right side, slowly bend the arm until the right palm is facing the right shoulder (close to the shoulder and right in front of it). Then the left arm tries to force the right back to the starting position while the right arm resists. Repeat with left arm. * See 60-Second Exercise Solution Guidelines.

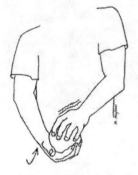

bottom arm curls up to shoulder
while top arm resists

closer arm is pushing
and outside arm resists
while being straightened

4. The Leg Extensions and Curls Sans Machines (strengthens the upper leg muscles — quadriceps and hamstrings)

Seated in a straight-back chair, cross the ankles with the left on top of the right. Start with the ankles/feet on the floor, directly under the front edge of the chair, and straighten the right leg while resisting with the left or top leg. When the legs are fully extended, reverse and have the left leg force the right back down to the starting position. Repeat with right on top of left. * See 60-Second Exercise Solution Guidelines.

inside leg straightens while
outside leg resists until legs
are straight

top leg pulls down
while bottom leg resists
until legs are bent and feet
are on floor just in front of chair

M. Mayhew

M. Mayhew

5. The Machine-less Seated Heel Raises (strengthens calf muscles)

Sit on the front edge of chair, with the knee of the left leg bent at a 90 degree angle and the foot directly under the knee. For best results, put a book or two down (making an approximately 3-inch high ledge or step) for the ball of the left foot to rest upon, with the heel unsupported. Slowly raise the heel by pressing the toes into the books while both hands push down on the left leg near the the knee for resistance. Then, reverse and with your hands pushing on the left leg near the knee try to push the heel back down (as it resists) until it is close to the floor in the starting position. Repeat with right leg. * See 60-Second Exercise Solution Guidelines.

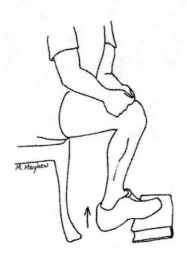 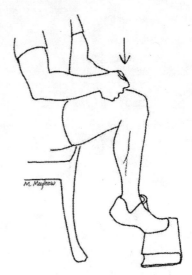

A. heel raises while arms resist   B. then arms push down while heel resists

6. Crunches (strengthens abdominal muscles)

Lie on back on the floor (a padded surface such as a rug) with the knees bent, feet flat on the floor. Put one hand under the head *to support* the neck and place the other hand on the stomach (or fold arms across the chest, as pictured). Lift the upper body off the floor just far enough for the shoulder blades to be airborne (about 3 to 6 inches); squeezing the abdominal muscles tightly. Slowly return back to floor. Repeat this process 10 times or until tired. Then raise up one more time and hold in this up position for a slow count of 10 (about 10 seconds) while squeezing the abs tightly (use the hand on the belly to check for tightness). Each week add 1 more crunch until you are doing about 20; also, add 1 more second to the held crunch at the end. Work up to 3 sets of 20 crunches and 3 sets of 20-second held crunches with 5 to 10 second rest periods in between sets. Optional: A more difficult (and rewarding) crunch is done with the feet off the ground and the shins parallel to the ground and simultaneously lifting the shoulder blades and the hips off the floor just slightly.

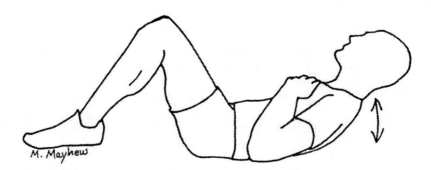

M. Mayhew

Fast Or Slow — Which way To Go?

Payton Jordan, the fastest human at various ages including 55 and 81 (11.6 seconds and 14.52 seconds respectively in the 100-meter sprint) used interval training to maintain his amazing speed through the years. For example, during workouts, he would run four 100-meter sprints at 16-18 seconds each, interspersed with 100-meter walks; and two 200-meter runs at 30 to 32 seconds each, with 200-meter jogs sandwiched in between the sprints. Watch young children and animals and you'll often see bursts of energy and action interlaced with periods of relative calm. It's a fun and natural way to get in one's aerobic workout in less time and with greater benefits and more smile per mile.

We don't last long exercising intensely, and so we jog or walk along at a slow, steady pace for our 30 or 40 minutes or more. If we were to go as hard as we could, we know we wouldn't last long enough to get any aerobic benefits and we might even injure ourselves. However, there is a third option; one in which we alternate the fast and slow. Bursts of energetic movement alternated with more moderate or slow movement allows us to exercise long enough to reap the aerobic rewards while allowing us to recapture some of the joy and exuberance of our youth.

Research published in the *Journal of Medicine and Science In Sports and Exercise* showed that when compared to low-intensity, long-duration exercise, high-intensity, interval training increased the number of calories burned in the hour after the exercise by a whopping 143%. This increase in metabolism (read, fat burning) lasts up to three hours after an interval workout.

Aerobic workouts using interval training can last from 10 to 40 minutes. As training for sports competition, it could last longer. More than 45 to 60 minutes would probably tear down our fitness and health rather than building it up. If, after an intense workout, you find yourself exhausted the next day and/or your resting pulse rate is around 10 beats above normal, then you may benefit from shorter workouts. Quality is more important than quantity. So what does any of this have to do with the 60-Second Solution?

The 60-Second Aerobic Solution #1

1. Spend the first 25 to 33 percent of an aerobic workout walking or jogging easily to warm up. Never stretch first; stretching "cold" muscles is more likely to cause injury than to prevent it. A recent study found that stretching before exercise actually weakens the muscles for about 15 minutes. The best time to stretch is at the end of a workout for general flexibility and for more limber muscles for future workouts; and perhaps after warming up to prepare for a high intensity workout.
2. Once properly warmed up, speed up by walking faster, jogging or sprinting (whichever is commensurate with your fitness level) for 15 to 60 seconds. You can do this on foot, bike, skates, treadmill, etc. Remember, it is better to undertrain in the beginning than to overdo and get sick or injured and lose your impetus
3. Walk or jog for 60 seconds.
4. Walk faster, jog or sprint for 15 to 60 seconds.
5. Continue this pattern of speeding up and slowing down for about 5 minutes at first. Over the course of weeks or months (whats the hurry?) increase the interval-training section of your workout to about 15 to 20 minutes (excludes warm-up and cool-down time). If done intensely enough, this is more than sufficient for just about *anyone* (and that definitely includes us).
6. Warm down or cool down (you get to choose the terminology) by walking or slow-running-followed-by-walking for 25 to 33 percent of your total exercise session.
7. *Gently* stretch out your muscles. If you are not sure what to do, procure a book or video and learn how to stretch properly, whether it is yoga or sports flexibility exercises.

The 60-Second Aerobic Solution #2

Here's a fun and effective variation:

1. Warm up with a 5-to-10-minute walk or until you feel warmed up.

2. Jog, run or sprint (i.e., increase intensity) for one minute.
3. Walk (i.e., decrease intensity) for 60 seconds.
4. Jog, run or sprint for two minutes.
5. Walk for 60 seconds.
6. Jog, run or sprint for three minutes.
7. Walk for 60 seconds.
8. Jog, run or sprint for two minutes.
9. Walk for 60 seconds.
10. Jog, run or sprint for one minute.
    Optional: Repeat this pattern (steps 2 through 10) one more time. Swimming, skating, rope jumping, stair-stepping, etc. may be enjoyed in place of the walk/run option.
11. Cool down by walking for 5 to 10 minutes or until you feel cooled down.

The 60-Second Desk-Workout Solution

Every hour or two, to be more productive, take a refreshing exercise break. **First**, stretch arms up toward the ceiling (really reaching) while taking in a deep breath; then relax as you exhale slowly while lowering arms. Do three times. Good for countering that bent-over-your-desk stress and tension. **Second**, sit on the edge of chair and lean slightly forward; stand up and sit down slowly 10 consecutive times without pushing off desk or chair arm rests in order to get up; over the ensuing weeks, work up to 25 times (if your chair is on castor wheels, make sure it hasn't rolled away between your seventh get-up and your seventh — whoops! — where can I find a foam donut?) If this is too easy, try one leg at a time. Eventually you can sneak a 10 to 25-pound weight plate under your desk for holding while you perform this effective leg strengthener. **Third**, every other workout, trade in the Stand-Ups for the old stand-by, push-ups. If others laugh, just think of yourself as a stand-up comedian with a smaller audience. **Fourth**, during phone calls, in standing position, rise up and down on toes/ball of one foot and then the other, while holding on to the back of a chair for balance (this is one of June Tatro's techniques for staying young and limber).

The 60-Second Tension-Release Solution

Sitting in a chair, lift feet off the floor, take a deep breath, and then tense every muscle in your body (including clenching the jaw, squinting the eyes, and curling the toes, etc.) while holding the breath to a slow count to 10. Slowly exhaling, relax every part of body while sinking down into chair. Repeat two more times. Then savor the new, relaxed feeling for a few moments (this is another of June's suggestions for a long, healthy life).

The 60-Second Stretching Solution

During Jerry Dunn's marathon of marathons, Jerry did virtually no stretching whatsoever. After each run he would go back to his car, get in and drive back to his motel.

Dr. Philip Maffetone helps train some of the world's elite athletes. One such athlete is Mark Allen, who won the Hawaiian Ironman Triathlon six times. Mr. Allen has said that he used Maffetone's workout structure during his competitive years. So what does Dr. Maffetone have to say about stretching? In his book, *The Maffetone Method*, he says that based on his experience in working with world-class athletes and beginners alike, most of us do not need to stretch if we warm up and cool down properly. As a matter of fact, he's found that those who stretch experience more injuries than those who don't.

I would suggest that you research the matter for yourself (this topic is beyond the scope of this book). If you are going to stretch, find an up-to-date book and/or video or two and learn how to stretch safely and effectively. Another option is to join a yoga/Tai-Chi class, or get a personal trainer from whom you can learn proper technique. If you are planning on competing in a sports event where a wide range of motion is called for or abrupt stops and turns are required, then proper stretching may indeed be imperative. However, if you are just planning to take long walks or jog, then the need is not quite so clear. Finally, recent studies have shown that gentle stretching after a strength-training workout, or after each set in a resistance workout, can actually increase strength gains.

The 60-Second Solution isn't enough for you? Check out the next chapter for programs that work.

CHAPTER 8 EIGHT THAT WORK

Many programs will work to create fit individuals. Some are more efficient and better designed than others. Some are easier to stick with over the long haul. The secret is to find a program that is fundamentally sound; that's built on the latest scientific understanding of what supports good health and fitness. Just as critical is to find a system that fits your needs, interest and personality. Our fitness champions were successful in getting ultra fit because they chose a vehicle that suited them best, one that motivated them to take action: for some it was running; for others it was swimming or biking; yet others turned to strength training. Likewise, they each chose nutritious diets, but each champion's diet is unique to his/her individual likes and dislikes.

Most of our Masters of Fitness started running, biking, swimming and lifting weights first, and then turned to books and other runners, swimmers, and weightlifters for motivation, support and proper technique. By joining running and biking clubs and getting personal trainers, coaches or training partners, they learned what they needed to know to get more and more fit and competitive. One of these programs that follow, and its author/creator, can act as your "coach" — an expert who can guide you to getting fitter after 50.

Some of the descriptions of these programs contain information about individuals and studies that were presented in earlier chapters and is being repeated here for your convenience and to better explain the effectiveness of these eight programs.

1. Strong Women Stay Young
(includes a program for men)

Overview - A fitness program focused on strength training for women and grounded in the sound research done at the world-famous Tufts University Center on Aging.

Who - Miriam E. Nelson, Ph.D., and/or her colleagues at the Tufts Center on Aging carried out extensive studies that showed that older adults can greatly benefit from high-intensity strength training. Most adults after age 35 or so start losing muscle and bone while adding fat. Some scientists think this is a major reason we slow down as we get older and get frail and feeble.

Does It Work? - In one study, Dr. Nelson had 40 post-menopausal women strength-train for one year. She and her associates then compared the strength-trained women with a non-exercising control group. The ST women gained muscle, bone mass and confidence, while the controls lost a little bit of all three. According to Dr. Nelson, the strength-trained individuals, based on post-tests, were 15 to 20 years younger biologically. In addition, women (and some men) who follow the *Strong Women Stay Young* program are continually citing their anecdotal success stories on the SWSY website and in Dr. Nelson's books. For instance, a 66-year-old woman who participated in aerobics classes three times per week and walked an hour a day on most other days wrote that she was surprised to be diagnosed with osteopenia. She continued the SWSY program and after one and one-half years her bone-density test results were back to normal.

Exercise Component - The SWSYP consists of two 30-minute strength-training sessions per week and recommends 30 minutes of aerobic activity (i.e., stair-climbing, walks, jogs, cycling, ...) on the other days. Just about everything a novice would need to know to get started building strength is included in the SWSY books and website. The program consists of eight strength exercises done in two sets of eight repetitions each. There is a program designed for home use and one for the gym.

Diet Component - Dr. Nelson recommends eating a balanced diet by following the United States Department of Agriculture's Food Guide Pyramid. This mainstream pyramid tells us how many servings of grains, fruits, etc. we should have each day. Dr. Nelson cautions us to watch the size of our servings because Americans tend to eat helpings that are much larger than what is recommended. This can lead to the unnecessary packing on of flab. For example, an "official" USDA serving of lean meat or fish is only 2 to 3 ounces (obviously, a 12-ounce T-bone would be four to six *times* larger) and a serving of vegetables is usually only one-half cup — so along with your knife and fork you may want to include a magnifying glass. Eight glasses of water each day is also encouraged. Vitamin supplements however, including protein powders for building muscle, are seen as unnecessary.

Other Components - Some of the shared research shows the tremendous benefits of strength training for even the frailest of the elderly. These benefits include regaining the ability to get out of a chair, walk without a cane or walker, and live independently. Also included is research showing strength training as invaluable in dealing with diabetes, osteoporosis, arthritis and heart disease. In addition, SWSY provides techniques for staying motivated and on track and answers many questions that may arise as we plan to start a strength-building program.

Strong Points - An excellent strength-building program for mature folks like us, based on solid research with older adults. Good, easy-to-follow directions and illustrations provided. Overall, an inexpensive and easy-to-follow scientifically-proven system.

Weak Points- Not really for men (thus the title, Strong *Women* Stay Young) or those who want more advanced/intense strength training. Only touches on aerobics and diet. Doesn't elaborate on the research enough for my tastes and interests.

For More Information:
Strong Women Stay Young, Miriam E. Nelson, Ph.D.
Strong Women Stay Slim, Miriam E. Nelson
WWW.StrongWomen.com

2. Body For Life Challenge

Overview - Body for Life is a strength-building program that promises to transform our body and life in just 12 weeks.

Who - BFL is the brainchild of Bill Phillips, a thirty-something bodybuilder, who founded Muscle Media Magazine and EAS, a leading bodybuilding supplement company. Mr. Phillips has an excellent track record; he has helped elite athletes such as Terrell Davis, John Elway, Karl Malone and Mike Piazza and hundreds of thousands of others (just like you and me) by answering their fitness and training questions and providing solutions.

Does It Work? - Al Cole, 52-year-old senior editor of *Modern Maturity* magazine (an AARP publication) and his wife Linda took the BFL challenge and reported their results, pictures and all, in a multi-page article in MM magazine. They reported dropping their cholesterol, blood pressure, and waist sizes significantly. Al's percentage of body fat went from 24.4 to 9.7; while Linda's shrank from from 26.3 to a svelte 14.0.

You may recall from chapter 3, seventy-two-year-old Daniel Weidner was recovering from a motorcycle accident when he discovered Body-For -Life. Following the BFL regimen, he added 15 pounds of lean body mass while shrinking his waist from 34 to 32 inches. He also increased his chest measurement from 33 inches to 38, and his biceps from 12 to 14.5 inches. As a result of his progress on this program, he was planning a 3,000-mile bicycle trip from New Jersey to California.

Larry Patrick, at age 57, had been suffering from clinical depression for seven long years when he decided to take the Body-For-Life Challenge. In just a few short months, using this system, he was able to reduce his 257-pound body from 27 percent bodyfat to a svelte 10 percent. He became a Body-For-Life champion, won $100,000, and oh yes, his depression lifted, too. *Muscle Media* magazine has before-and-after pictures and stories galore of others who have had similar transformations.

Exercise Component - There are three strength and three aerobic workouts a week with one day off. The strength workouts alternate between Upper Body and Lower Body and last approximately 47 minutes (UB) and 38 minutes (LB). The aerobic sessions are just 20 minutes of intense-interval training each. BFL is built around the idea that more is not necessarily better; high-quality, high-intensity training is superior.

Diet Component - Six nutritious mini-meals each day are the centerpiece of the BFL diet. It is highly recommended that each meal contain a complex carbohydrate (e.g., rice, a sweet potato, potato, oatmeal, etc.) and a protein source (e.g., salmon, chicken, lean beef, tofu, etc.) with both helpings the size of the individual's fist. Several of the meals include a vegetable or two or fruit. The meals are low fat with fat grams counted and severely limited. One day a week is set aside to eat anything that is desired. Oh yes, there is a slew of body-building supplements to choose from and take (i.e., protein powders, creatine, meal replacements, fat-burners, etc.).

Other Components - For motivation, there is a million-dollar, 12-week Body For Life challenge/bodybuilding contest sponsored by EAS. This includes inspirational videos of success stories, gobs of before-and-after pictures of everyday folk, instruction in how to stay "pumped" (i.e., excited) and prizes/prize money galore.

Strong Points - Plenty of examples of those who have made remarkable transformations with the BFL system abound to fortify your belief that you, too, can do this. Every detail from exercise charts to record one's progress to before-and-after photo session instructions, to menus and recipes for the six meals/day has been worked out for you. There is also a ten issue-per-year magazine, *Muscle Media*, to keep you up to speed, inspired and help you deal with the inevitable obstacles. Incredibly, the workouts only total about three hours per week.

Weak Points - This program is basically for strength and body-building. It's not the best choice for those who would much rather get the bulk of their exercise in some aerobic form, such as long distance biking or swimming. Also, the supplements which are a requirement for the contest, but not for following the BFL protocol, require a hefty investment.

> **For More Information:**
> www.BodyForLife.com
> *Muscle Media* magazine
> *Body For Life* by Bill Phillips. Harper Collins Publisher: New York, NY, 1999.

3. The McDougall Plan

Overview - The McDougall Program promises just 12 days to dynamic health, and it delivers. Its main tenet is that our diet is at the root of a host of diseases and that for dramatic changes in one's health, dramatic dietary and lifestyle changes are needed

Who - According to Dean Ornish, M.D., (the doctor who proved that heart disease can be reversed), "Dr. John McDougall, M.D., is a true pioneer in using low-fat, vegetarian diets to treat and help prevent a variety of diseases." McDougall runs his program out of the St. Helena Hospital and Health Center in California and claims that in 12 years of treating heart patients, all his patients who have adopted a healthy-heart diet have avoided surgery.

Does It Work? In 1999 a major insurance company carefully studied his regimen for improving health. For six weeks they followed 13 of his typical patients and found these startling results:

1. Ninety health conditions were solved without medical intervention.
2. Thirty-one drugs were discontinued.
3. Each person was projected to save an average of $2,389 per year ($1,589.52 saved on prescription drugs alone).

In his book, *The McDougall Program,* he gives a detailed 12-day log/progress report on two patients, a husband and wife. This account includes their before, during and after-lab reports/blood work. The husband had angina pain when he started (which was also the reason he turned to Dr. McDougall for help), was on several medications (including Dyazide, Inderal and Nitroglycerin tablets), and could only walk 5 or 10 minutes at a time, stopping frequently due to chest pains. By the twelfth day he had no chest pains, was taking two 30-minute walks per day, and was off all the medications. Both he and his wife had significant improvements in their weight, cholesterol, triglycerides and blood-sugar levels.

A year later they were still on the program and his blood pressure was down from 158/104 to 110/70; his weight had plummeted from 213 pounds to 170; his cholesterol drop was 246 mg/dl to 138; and his triglycerides went from 275 mg/dl to 130. The wife's numbers were impressive, too. These included an improvement in weight from 135 to 115; cholesterol from 218 to 124; and her blood sugar had gone from 98 to 78. With their newfound youthfulness, they were now enjoying walking, hiking, swimming and skiing. I'll grant that this is all reported from the good doctor's perspective, but it would be impressive even if it were only partially true.

Exercise Component - This program is centered around making dietary changes. As far as exercise is concerned, his recommendation is to get some mild-to-moderate exercise every day ... for instance, 30-minute walks once or twice a day.

Diet Component - As a young doctor serving the workers on sugar cane plantations, Dr. McDougall noticed that the older generations of Japanese, Chinese, and Philipino workers were, almost without exception, healthy and robust into their seventh, eighth and ninth decade of life. Meanwhile, the younger generations of workers (doing the same work), who had adopted an Americanized diet high in refined sugar, fatty meats, and dairy products, were very sickly in comparison. Diabetes, high blood pressure, heart disease and obesity were rampant in the younger adult workers and almost nonexistant in their elders. Through his years of research, McDougall came to the conclusion that diet is the primary causative factor in about 34 different diseases.

The McDougall dietary plan centers around starches (e.g., sweet potatoes, rice, oatmeal, ...) with plenty of fresh or frozen fruits and vegetables thrown in. His diet eliminates meats, dairy products, eggs, oils and other rich foods except during rare, special events like weddings, graduations and holidays.

Other Components - This plan can be followed at home or at the St. Helena Hospital and Health Center where for several days temptation can be kept to a minimum while the client comes to the realization that this new lifestyle really does work and is worth it.

Strong Points - The McDougall program has a proven track record. If you were to go to the center, you would have the finest medical attention, including ongoing lab tests to keep you and the medical staff apprised of your progress. Also, you have the option of going it alone in the comfort of your own home. There are easy-to-prepare, delicious recipes and menus to help you make the transition from a typical American diet to a more healthful, possibly medication-reducing fare. For those who despise exercise, this is a good program because the exercise component is so minimal.

Weak Points - Low fat diets such as this are typically difficult to stick with given our society's culinary temptations and considering how tasty fatty foods can be. However, if you have serious health issues, then this may be the answer for you. On the other hand, if you don't have a compelling reason to go this route, then a more moderate diet with a more significant role for exercise may be more suited to your needs and desires.

For More Information:
www.DrMcDougall.com
The McDougall Program, John A. McDougall, M.D.

4. The Cooper Wellness Program

Overview - The non-profit Cooper Aerobics Center is a multi-divisional health and fitness complex that is dedicated to advancing the understanding of the relationship between living habits and health. It promotes a balanced approach that includes diet, exercise, stress management and health/fitness assessments based on the latest research (much of which they do themselves at the Cooper Institute).

Who - Kenneth H. Cooper, M.D., the president and founder of the Cooper Aerobics Institute in Dallas and the "father of Aerobics," believes that "it is easier to maintain good health through proper exercise, diet, and emotional balance than to regain it once it is lost." His institute has been a world leader in fitness research and education since 1970.

Does It Work? Doctors and researchers at the Cooper Aerobics Center have shown that moderate activity (such as that which they include in their wellness program) reduces deaths from cancer, diabetes, heart disease and strokes by 55 percent and significantly prolongs life. Professional and elite amateur athletes, movie stars, and politicians from around the world have been descending on the Center for almost 30 years now to have their fitness level analyzed and to seek expert guidance — so they must be doing something right. This is where Helen Klein came to have her fitness and health analyzed. In her mid-seventies at the time, her heart and lungs were assessed to be commensurate to a 30-year-old's and antioxidants were prescribed to keep it so.

Exercise Component - A leader in fitness research, the Cooper Institute recommends a program of walking, jogging, cycling or some other aerobic activity at least three or four times per week, 20 to 30 minutes per session. In the beginning their focus was just on aerobics, but in recent years they've discovered the importance of balancing aerobic training with strength training. Because we tend to lose muscle mass as we get older, they promote a program of increasing the strength component as we age. For someone in his/her thirties, they recommend a workout consisting of about 80 percent aerobic to 20 percent strength. Over the years, this program ideally shifts emphasis, so that by age sixty, the workout has become 55 percent aerobic and 45 percent strength. Walk For Life is a

12-week program they have developed for beginners. It gives novices a step-by-step, safe means of getting fit.

Diet Component - The Cooper Institute's emphasis is on a balanced, nutritious diet with plenty of whole grains, fruits and vegetables to stay healthy and reduce the risk of cancer and heart disease. A balance of carbohydrates (more complex carbs than simple sugars), proteins, and fats is promoted. On the fat front they would have you keep your saturated (animal) fats to a minimum while getting more monounsaturated fats in the form of olive and canola oils; and acquiring omega-3's from deep-sea fish, nuts and seeds. They also recommend 6 to 8 glasses of water per day and antioxidant-rich foods and supplements.

Other Components - They offer a clinical Weight Management Center, Scientific Update/Conferences, and a comprehensive Lifestyle Training/Medical Spa Program. There are 4-day and one or two-week stays at the 30-acre campus for lifestyle modification training and personalized fitness assessments. Programs and amenities include relaxation training, nutritional counseling, gourmet meals, use of spa and massage services (not exactly a boot-camp experience) and more.

Strong Points - The Cooper Institute does its own world-class research and bases its programs and services on their findings and the latest medical findings of other researchers (i.e., sound science). One can follow its programs at home or travel to Dallas for a first-class fitness/spa experience.

Weak Points - As a respected leader in preventive-medicine research and education, The Cooper Institute has to protect its hard-earned reputation by being a bit conservative in their recommendations. In other words, it does not want to risk its standing in the health/medical community by promoting a cutting-edge technique or program that later turns out to be bogus or dangerous. If you want the latest innovations and programs in the fitness arena, you'll have to go elsewhere.

For More Information:
www.CooperAerobics.com
www.CooperAerobics.com/tip_WalkForLife.htm
Dr. Kenneth H. Cooper's Antioxidant Revolution,
Can Stress Heal? Kenneth H. Cooper, M.D.

5. The Maffetone Method

Overview - According to Dr. Maffetone this is a program for fitness *and* health (he differentiates between the two) that one can and will stick with for life. He bills it as a holistic, low-stress, no-pain way to exceptional fitness. This plan centers around aerobic training while emphasizing a balance between aerobic and anaerobic activities. The good doctor defines aerobic as using body fat, instead of sugar, as one's energy source.

Who - Dr. Philip Maffetone has practiced complementary sports medicine for over 20 years, during which time he has trained many world-class athletes, as well as thousands of us normal folk. He is one of the most sought-after endurance coaches/trainers in the world.

Does It Work? Triathlete Mark Allen used Maffetone's workout structure to train for and win 6 Hawaiian Ironman Triathlons. Now that his competitive days are over, he continues to use these training principles to stay fit for life.

One-thousand-mile world champion, Stu Mittleman, was trained by Dr. Maffetone. It took Mittleman just over 11 days to complete this insane footrace; a fascinating and very significant footnote to this feat is that at the end of this exercise in perpetual motion, Mittleman looked better and felt stronger than when he started. Maffetone also trained the Canadian champion of the thousand-miler. Obviously Dr. Maffetone's fitness strategies work and we can learn much about building our endurance for life from him.

Exercise Component - The Maffetone Method says that:

1. The best form of exercise for good health and burning fat is an aerobic activity, such as walking, running, swimming, dancing, ...
2. Exercise should be fun. If it is not, you are working out too intensely; or your sessions are too long; or your training partner is more of a hindrance than a help.
3. Exercise can relieve stress or add to it depending on how it is done.
4. Always warm up and cool down. In aerobic training this does not necessarily mean including stretching (which may cause more injuries than it prevents).

5. If you are unsure of how to start or what to do, just commence walking several times per week.
   Diet Component -
1. Drink at least six 8-ounce glasses of water each day. Coffee, sodas, juices and other beverages are not a substitute for clean, pure water.
2. Avoid foods that are sugar laden, such as cookies, cakes, pies and candies.
3. Stay away from foods that contain hydrogenated and partially hydrogenated fats.
4. Eliminate white-flour products from your diet.
5. Eat at least four to six servings of cooked vegetables in a rainbow of colors each day, and one or more raw vegetables (sound familiar?).
6. "Good" dietary fats can actually help you to burn more bodyfat and stay healthy.
7. Chew your food well and eat in a relaxed atmosphere.

All these 7 seven steps are for the purpose of changing us from sugar-burners into fat-burning machines.

Other Components - Dr. Maffetone recommends using a heart-rate monitor, his formula, and his Maximum Aerobic Function Test to find our maximum aerobic heart rate. This test involves calculating the time it takes to travel (by running, biking, swimming, ...) a set distance and monitoring our heart rate during the test. From this information we determine our aerobic training zone — our fat-burning zone. Another integral part of this method is stress management.

Strong Points - Exercising in one's aerobic training zone is very comfortable. It makes exercising easy and fun for just about anyone. It may seem wimpy at first to the competitor in us, but it has proven itself time and again in building an aerobic base upon which ultimate athletic success is built.

Weak Points - Those who use Maffetone's MAF (Maximum Aerobic Function) and Aerobic Training Zone for the first time may find the exercise seems too easy. That is, most of us don't like how slowly we have to move in order to to keep our heart rate in the aerobic training zone. I didn't.

The program starts with building an aerobic base (i.e., our aerobic/endurance fitness). During this time, which can last from three to five months — sometimes longer — no anaerobic training is allowed. That means no interval training, racing, or hard, challenging training runs. This can be a downer for those of us who love our anaerobic workouts.

For More Information:

The Maffetone Method, Dr. Philip Maffetone, Ragged Mountain Press/McGraw-Hill
www.RaggedMountainPress.com
Slow Burn, Stu Mittleman, Harper Collins (a similar program by a Maffetone protégé)

6. HeartMath Stress-Management Techniques

Overview - A series of stress management techniques that can be used almost anywhere/anytime to make us fitter after 50 and biologically younger.

The heart generates the strongest electromagnetic field produced by the body (over 5,000 times more powerful than that of the brain) and radiates this signal to all that individual's other organs and systems (such as, the lungs and the immune system). When the heart's rhythm is incoherent, as it is whenever we are experiencing any negative emotions, it sends a distress signal to the rest of the body, thereby putting the whole body on a collision course with catabolism. When the heart's signal is coherent, the rest of the body's systems, including the nervous system and brain, entrain with the heart's electromagnetic field, resulting in laser-beam-like efficiency, the elimination of excess stress, and a youthful anabolic state. The HeartMath's mental/emotional techniques focus positive thoughts and emotions around the heart, producing coherent heart signals. Over time, the result is a fitter, more youthful you.

Who - The Institute of HeartMath in Boulder Creek, California was founded by Doc Lew Childre. It is known for its stress-reduction seminars and its cutting-edge research. Prestigious medical journals, such as the American Journal of Cardiology and the Journal of Advancement In Medicine, have published IHM research papers.

Does It Work? A study was conducted at the Motorola Corporation's Florida plant. At the beginning of the study, 25 percent of the participating employees were found to have high blood pressure. After six months of instruction in and

212

practice of the HeartMath stress-reduction techniques, all the employees had normal blood-pressure levels without conventional medical intervention.

In other IHM research involving 45 healthy adults, after just one month of practicing HeartMath techniques, the test subjects had raised their DHEA (dehydroepiandrosterone — "the fountain of youth hormone") by an average of 100 percent and decreased their cortisol (the "stress hormone") by 23 percent. DHEA typically peaks in adolescence and then starts a steady decline as we age. It is significant that the precursor to many other hormones, including testosterone, estrogen, progesterone and human growth hormone, is DHEA. Scientists are finding a close correlation between low levels of DHEA and Alzheimer's disease, obesity, diabetes, cardiovascular disease and other maladies usually associated with aging.

Joseph Chilton Pearce, author of *Evolution's End*, suffered from severe tachycardia, arrhythmia and atrial fibrillation. Now in robust health again, he credits the HeartMath techniques with giving him back his life and getting him off his dependency on heart medications.

I, myself, have experienced these life-enhancing techniques. I have practiced these methods while hooked up to a heart-rate monitor and have seen their effectiveness displayed on the computer screen.

Exercise Component - None

Diet Component - None

Other Components - The Institute of HeartMath offers scientifically-designed music that has been shown to raise one's levels of the anti-aging hormone, DHEA, when used in combination with their emotional stress-management methods. They also have retreats and seminars where one can learn the techniques and the science behind them. A third component is their computer hardware/software, produced for independent training in, and practice of, their anabolism-promoting techniques.

Strong Points - For those who don't want to rely on exercise or change their eating habits, here is a way to increase anti-aging hormones using mental techniques. There are no vitamins to buy, no trips to the local health-food store, and no exhausting workouts. These techniques, once we learn them, are free (seminars, books, tapes, ... will take an investment) and can be used almost anywhere/anytime. Of course the IHM staff would want us to know that they are even more effective when combined with other healthful lifestyle choices, such as exercise and a quality diet.

Weak Points - Although the books and tapes are reasonably priced, some of the products/events/training are what some would call expensive. However, it's a first-class organization with five-star-rated seminars, retreats and training sessions, and as they say, "you get what you pay for."

For More Information:
www.HeartMath.org
Freeze-Frame, Doc Lew Childre
Cut Thru, Doc Lew Childre

7. The Spark

Overview - A 3-week fitness plan that emphasizes short, manageable, bite-size exercise sessions and a doable diet tailored to individual needs and lifestyle.

Who - Dr. Glenn A. Gaessar, University of Virginia, bases this very convenient and realistic (fits nicely into our modern, hectic lifestyle) program on his ground-breaking Spark Study 2000 research. His co-author, Karla Dougherty, adds spice as she tells of her metamorphosis from certifiable couch potato to marathon bicyclist at age — you guessed it — 50.

Does It Work? In only 3 weeks, the 40 participants in the Spark Study, averaged:

1. A 10-to-15 percent improvement in aerobic capacity (equivalent to a person 10 to 15 years younger).
2. A 40-to-100 percent increase in muscular endurance and strength (In other words, they were now biologically 20 years younger).
3. A "20-year" improvement in flexibility.
4. Significant decreases in blood levels of cholesterol, "evil" LDL cholesterol and triglycerides.
5. A comfortable, safe one-pound loss per week.

Exercise Component - This highly-effective exercise program is designed to fit into anyone's busy schedule by breaking up two and one-half hours of exercise per week into fifteen 10-minute sessions. This includes seven to ten aerobic workouts; two to four strength sessions; and two to four flexibilty Sparks. That's just two or three short-exercise bouts per day. For instance, one could park away from the office in the morning and take a 10-minute walk to work; do some push-ups and crunches at lunch time; and play soccer or tag with the kids at night.

Diet Component - The Spark program has just one diet rule, eat more fiber. Over three weeks, one *gradually* increases his/her diet's fiber content until it reaches 25 grams of fiber a day. A study published in the Journal of the American Medical Association in 1999 showed that those who ate the most fiber had the most success controlling their weight, no matter how many calories they consumed. The Spark food plan emphasizes fiber-rich complex carbohydrates — fruits, vegetables, whole grains, legumes, nuts and seeds.

Other suggestions include snacking often, but on nutritious foods. We are advised to watch our portion sizes. Having protein sources in our diet to build muscle, eating low-fat dairy, and drinking plenty of water are among other bits of advice.

Other Components - There are sample daily exercise schedules and menus for all 21 days for those who need every minute detail spelled out. Recipes are included and there is even an exercise log and a fiber log to keep track of our progress and keep us on track.

Strong Points - The 10-minute exercise segments are easy to fit into the busiest of schedules. The dietary changes/improvements are minimal and introduced gradually, as are the workouts. Changes are incorporated so gently/slowly that it most likely would minimize the muscle soreness and the injuries that so often derail overzealous, make-up-for-lost-years novices (also known as exercise drop-outs). Anyone who is serious about improving his/her fitness can follow this well-scripted plan and stick with it for years to come. And, nothing says we can't increase the length or number of workouts.

Weak Points - This plan is not for the serious athlete or fitness enthusiast, but is great for the beginner or those who have been sedentary for a while. The biggest complaint that I have is one of semantics. Glenn and Karla use the word "spark" and related words, such as "embers" and "kindling" so frequently that it made me want to torch the book before I lit a single exercise spark or enjoyed week one's embers or developed a burning desire to stoke my diet with some fiber sparks.

For More Information:
www.TheSparkPlan.com
The Spark, Dr. Glenn A. Gaessar and Karla Dougherty

8. Team Diabetes

Overview - This is an opportunity to join a team and get training to run or walk a marathon (or a shorter race) while raising money for a worthwhile cause. You get guaranteed entry in the marathon of your choice and free travel and accommodations for the marathon weekend. As I wrote this, some of the marathon choices were Walt Disney World, Rome City Marathon, Kona Hawaii Marathon, and Dublin City Marathon. What's the catch? You have to raise a minimum number of dollars or pesos, or ...

Who - The American Diabetes Association, with the help of corporate sponsors, offers this fundraiser and opportunity of a lifetime.

Does It Work? Our own Helen Klein was one of the Team Diabetes coaches for a while (now she and her husband Norm are coaching a middle school track team). Seasoned, professional coaches, like Helen, *can* train you to complete a marathon (running or walking). It's a gradual process of getting ready that takes about 6 months, but those who stick it out invariably have the thrill of running in and completing this potentially life-changing event.

Exercise Component - Whether you are an experienced marathoner or a beginner, you will receive the training and support that you need. You will be coached on form, training schedules to follow, and all aspects and intricacies of marathoning that you need to know. Team Diabetes will organize regular training runs or walks in your area. and teach you about cardiovascular endurance, flexibility, and weight control. You may even be able to choose a half-marathon or 10K race instead of a full marathon.

Diet Component - You will be advised on proper nutrition and hydration for before, during and after the marathon.

Other Components - Besides the "free" (if you get sufficient donations) travel and accomodations to one of the world's most beautiful travel destinations and well-known marathon courses (or a more local race), you will receive a comprehensive, individualized training plan designed by your coach. You also get a Team Diabetes T-shirt and race singlet. Finally, you will have the fun and camaraderie of being a member of Team Diabetes and helping in a worthy cause, and may even play a part in finding the cure.

Strong Points - It appears to be a win-win situation for all involved. It all sounds good to me, except for ...

Weak Points - If you live away from a major population area, you may have to travel to get to your team's training sessions, or you may have to get your coaching by E-mail or over the phone. Also, it will take some effort on your part to raise sufficient contributions to the Ameican Diabetes Association (for research, education, etc.) to make it worth their while to pay your way. You may consider this a positive or a negative, depending on your perspective.

For More Information:
www.Diabetes.org/TeamDiabetes/Team03/
1-888-DIABETES
1-888-342-2383

There are, of course, other good programs worth mentioning here:

Infinity2's Complete Physique is a good program. Its exercise component consists of super-slow strength-building exercises performed to a torturous 7/7 count (that can be done at home with a minimum of equipment). These exercises are so effective that a fitness expert and power lifter named Doug Grant used them in training to set a new world record of 125 push-ups in 60 seconds (Spring, 2001). The downside to these potent slo-mo workouts is that few people stick with them for long. These strength workouts are balanced with some aerobics, sound dietary recommendations, and supplementation centered around enzymes and probiotics. For more information, check out www.Infinity2.com or call 1-800-572-0501 to order *The Complete Physique* book.

Lance Armstrong, 3-time winner of the Tour de France, and his coach, Chris Carmichael, have a plan for the serious cyclists, from beginner to advanced. It's in book form, titled *The Lance Armstrong Performance Program.*

Then there's Tai chi (see Pat Rice's story in chapter 9), yoga (Helen Klein, 79, Gerry Davidson, 80, [Introduction], and Kathy Smart [next chapter] practice yoga to be limber for their other fitness-related pursuits) Pilates, spinning and on and on. Keep in mind that the most important aspect of all of this is finding something that fits your personality — a program that you will enjoy.

Young children are in constant motion; as we get older, many of us move less and less, until one day we stop moving altogether. There is a name for that; it's called being dead. Get moving for the fun of it; eat for the joy of it; and focus on what you like for the life-sustaining invigoration of it!

CHAPTER 9 FITTER AFTER 50 HITS HOME

Neither Mary nor Ed is a champion athlete by any stretch of the imagination, but they both are definitely fitter after 50. Here are their stories and those of eight local (Shenadoah Valley) fitness champions.

Ed's Story

I have always been interested in the topics of sports, fitness and health; and although exercise and working out have been a way of life since my youth, my personal bests in push-ups, pull-ups, the mile run, ... have come in my mid-fifties. How can a lifelong exerciser be fitter at age 56 than he has been at any other time? The answer resides in the wisdom of age. In my earlier years, I kept up a frenetic pace — always running, biking, exercising with some newfangled device, or playing some kind of ball. I was very active, but my "exercise" routines were extremely inefficient. There was no rhyme or reason, no well-thought-out plan. Relatively random movement and self-induced stress ruled my world. The stress was tearing down the muscle as fast as I could build it.

Through trial and error and a lifetime of experience, I have learned to get more out of less. Fewer workouts for more muscle. Shorter sessions and more rest for greater aerobic capacity. The secret is to work smarter; not just harder. Using the knowledge of those who have gone before me, those who have blazed a fitness trail, I have *finally* learned how to enjoy and benefit from the movements/activities of a well-thought-out plan.

Ed's Workout

Usually exercising less than four hours per week (an average of just over 30 minutes a day) has resulted in my being in the best shape of my life. Here's my routine:

Monday - 20 to 25-minute upper body & abdominal strength workout

Tuesday - 30-minute easy run/walk or bike ride

Wednesday - 30-minute run/walk interspersed with 3 or 4 sets of pull-ups

Thursday - 30-minute speed work on the track

>**Friday** - 40-minute upper, lower, & ab strength workout

>**Saturday** - Rest

>**Sunday** - One-hour to one-hour-twenty-minute 6 to 10-mile run

Personal Bests

The results of this very doable routine are several personal bests:

* 44 push-ups in 30 seconds at age 56
* 40 consecutive pull-ups at age 54
* 6:11 mile at age 56
* Resting pulse rate of 49 BPM at age 56
* Washboard Abs (you'll have to take my word for it)

These new personal bests take on even more significance when you know the rest of the story. First, I was never very good at push-ups and the most I can ever recall being able to do (even without a time restraint) was thirty-something. Forty-four in 30 seconds is quite an improvement, if I do say so myself.

Pull-ups have always been a favorite of mine ever since I was a kid with a chin-up bar permanently supported between two trees. As a student in junior high, I remember scoring well on this fitness test item — maybe doing 10 or 12 pull-ups. I continued to find bars and tree limbs on which to do chin-ups through the years, *always* counting how many I could do. One time in my mid-thirties, I achieved the significant (to me) score of 30 consecutive pull-ups. For the next 20 years I never came close to that record. Then at age 54, my friend Taylor and I took Bill Phillips' Body For Life body-building/transformation challenge. As a result of this program, we both gained muscle while losing fat. I gained about ten pounds of muscle while dropping two pounds of fat (I was under 160 pounds and didn't really have much fat to lose). During this 12-week challenge, I tied my record of 30 pull-ups; then a week later, it was 33; then 34, followed by 37; and finally, 40 pull-ups in a row. That's a 33 percent increase over my old record. Wow! Made my day. Now I can do 30 or more chin-ups just about every time I jump up to a chinning-bar, as long as I'm properly warmed up.

I have been a recreational jogger since my college days. In my mid-twenties, I timed myself at 6:15 for the mile. Not a great score, by any standards by which runners are ranked, but it was the best I had ever done, and would be for my next 30 years or so of running. During Phillips' challenge, one day on our neighborhood high school track, I tied my 6:15 score. I figured I could break it in the ensuing weeks, but it was not to be. Two years later, at age 56, my current age, I ran a 6:16 on the same track. It was very frustrating to come so close, but a hopeful sign at the same time. Then in July of 2001, I ran in the Loudon Street Mile (a local race). I wasn't expecting much, as I'd been painting our house that week, and my legs felt heavy and tight from all the time I had spent going up and down and precariously balancing on the ladder. At the quarter-mile, I had one minute and thirty-one seconds — a little fast, I thought. Better slow down. I didn't catch the times at the half-mile and three-quarter-mile markers, so I had no way of knowing how I was doing, as I am not an experienced miler who could recognize his pace. As I approached the finish line with a couple hundred yards to go, I looked at my watch and thought, "Oh, my gosh — golly-geewhiz, I could break my record." So I picked up the pace and sprinted past a pesky 12-year-old. As the time clock stared me in the face, I could see that I was going to set a new personal best, and did so with an *official* 6:11. It only took me 30 years to break my mile record. I have a feeling that I had better not wait another 30 to try to beat this mark, so I'll be back next year *sans* the painting gig and loaded for bear. I almost forgot: I received a second place trophy in my age group for my efforts. Plus, I was "walking on air" for the next couple of days.

5K and 10K Runs

There are running races of various distances almost every weekend, often within easy driving distance of wherever you are (unless you live in the middle of nowhere). I occasionally run in these friendly competitions, and have a couple of pertinent stories to tell you.

About twenty years ago, when I was in my thirties, the local community college sponsored an annual 5-mile race. I ran in it for a few years (my only race each year). One year I decided to train for it by bouncing on a small round trampoline called a rebounder. I had heard and read all the hype on this fad exercise gadget. It was supposed to be the best thing since swiss cheese, the best exercise one could possibly do to get in shape. I spent many an hour bouncing on this contraption in all sorts of contortions and often high enough to bang my head on the ceiling (not recommended for the ceiling or the head). I really thought this super exercise would do the trick, so I only ran two times in the months leading up to the 5-miler.

The day of the race I gave it my best shot on the rather hilly course, really pushing myself to get my best time. When I finished my usual sprint to the finish line, I was in bad shape. Feeling as if I could die right on the spot, I was too ill to even be embarrassed by having to have the paramedics lay me down and give me oxygen — the only runner to need such drastic measures. I learned the hard way the law of specificity; that is, for running races, one must practice running; for cycling, one must spend considerable time on a bike; and so forth. You can be the greatest runner in the world, but very little of that conditioning will transfer over to a swimming competition. Without the swimming training, the strongest of athletes will still struggle and sink to the bottom in a long swimming race. That's why swimmers swim almost exclusively and runners don't.

By age 54, I'd moved to a larger town with a longer race, an annual 10K. After a 15-year hiatus to catch my breath, I decided to tackle my first 10K. My 5-miler times had been around 37:30 or 7:30 per mile. Ten-K's are 6.2 miles, while 5-milers are — well, 5 miles. Therefore, when I ran my second 10K in 7:32 per mile, I knew that I was just about as fit as I'd been in my thirties. I was pleased!

In my most recent 10K, at age 56, I was once again up on my toes sprinting toward the finish, thinking that I was really flying, when a young stud I judged to be about 23 or 24-years-young passed me right at the finish line. I thought at the time that he was racing me, trying to beat yours truly. But when I checked the final standings in the newspaper a couple of days later, I found a 24-year-old lieutenant with a time just a second faster than mine AND yet another 24-year-old lieutenant with a time slightly slower than mine. Obviously, the military officers had been racing each other and I just happened to be between them. The relevant point to mull over is that a 56-year-old was right there with a couple of fit young servicemen at the end of 6.2 miles of racing. Yet, I only finished sixth among the 55-to-59 age group. There were about 720 competitors, 95 percent of them younger than I, yet I finished in the top one-third of these fittest of the fit. You see, we really can be fitter after 50.

Finally, a recent 5K race has an interesting subplot. As I neared the final stretch of the race, I spied two men in front of me. I decided that I might be able to catch them. With a furious kick I ended up with the same time as one of the men, 22:37 (7'17" per mile — my fastest 5K to date). This gentleman turned out to be 34 years old; I am 56 (remember?) He placed second in the 30-34 age group; I languished in fifth place in my age bracket. This is yet another reminder that we can be fitter after 50 — fitter than (or as fit as, to be precise) some thirty-year-olds, even fit ones.

Mary's Story

When we married in our early twenties, Ed and I had decided that health and fitness would be a life priority. The plan was to eliminate foods containing white flour and sugar (substituting honey and whole wheat flour in scratch recipes), to supplement our diets with vitamins and minerals, and to maintain an exercise regimen (I jogged about six miles a week). Although I was convinced that this plan was sufficient for optimal health, three things indicated that it was not: my lungs, my sinuses, and my looks.

My lungs literally complained. They were wheezy. Had I been diagnosed, a doctor might have deemed me mildly asthmatic; inhalations and exhalations were slow, labored, and noisy. Jogging regularly must have helped the situation a little, but not much, it seemed.

The sinus problem had been with me since childhood and followed me into adulthood. There was chronic sinus drainage; there were nasty, incapacitating infections and rhinitis, along with occasional colds and flu.

As for my looks, my body was soft looking. It spread and squished out too much, especially in the backside area. Youth was on my side, though. Although I was not overjoyed with my body, it could have been worse (and I did not realize it could

223

have been better), so the moderate jogging routine comprised my complete exercise program for about seventeen years.

Years have passed, and one by one, the problems have disappeared. Now, in my mid-fifties, I am the fittest I have ever been. Here is what I did:

* The sinus problem: Around age twenty-six, I eliminated red-meat from my diet (and we ate lots of it). A few months later, the chronic sinus drainage and flare-ups of infection stopped. I am still vegetarian (I do eat eggs, dairy, and occasional seafood); my sinuses remain clear and infection free. Rhinitis and colds are practically non-existent.

* The wheezy lung syndrome: After the birth of our second child, when I was about forty-one years old, I decided to gradually increase my jogging to five miles daily for five or six days a week. The lungs cleared. Even though I do not jog that much now, the lungs remain clear. Here is my modest (but effective) aerobic regimen:

1. Tuesdays and Thursdays I run at the high school track. I run a half mile to get there, run fast twice around, jog slowly 1/2 lap, run fast 1 1/2 laps, jog 1/2 lap, run fast one lap, jog 1/2 lap, run fast 1 1/2 laps, run up about 75 high school front steps, and then run the half mile home.
2. Sundays: Ed and I run together for ten kilometers (6.2 miles) cross-country at my [slower] pace... about an hour.

* The "squishy" body? Gone! How? Two things:

1. Weight training! For years I had resisted Ed's suggestion to do moderate weight training. Aerobics, I insisted, was enough. Then, in our early fifties, Ed bought a small piece of exercise equipment called the "Total Gym," which converted me into a believer! At my request, Ed chose some exercises for me from the Total Gym instruction booklet which take about 20-30 minutes to do and alternately strengthen the upper and lower-body muscle systems. There are 11 exercises which strengthen every significant

muscle group in the upper body, and five exercises to tighten thighs and tummy. I do these sets alternately every Monday, Wednesday, and Friday. That is, upper-body workouts on Monday and Friday with a lower-body session on Wednesday one week — lower-body workouts on Monday and Friday (upper body Wednesday) the next week.

Before each of these training sessions (all three days), I strengthen and tighten the derriere with the following *very effective* exercise: I have fashioned a weight by threading a lightweight rope through two doughnut-shaped 4.4-pound weights and tying the ends, leaving enough slack to put my foot through so the resulting 8.8-pound weight could dangle from my ankle. Holding onto a chairback to steady myself, standing on one foot and holding the weighted leg straight behind me, I lift the weight off the floor slowly for 28 or 30 repetitions. I repeat with the other leg. The gluteal muscles get a great workout. I also lift the weight 28-30 times a little to the side (about "4 o'clock") to tighten the muscles in the "saddlebag" area. After each series of 28-30 lifts, I hold the weighted leg up for another count of 28 or 30. This exercise, combined with one more thing, has done more to tame the "outback" than any other.

2. The "one more thing": Lipochromizyme! I am not being paid or otherwise cajoled to endorse any products here, but when I find an outstanding one, I will recommend it without apology. The one which has made a big difference in the success of my exercise program is Lipochromizyme, from the Infinity2 (Infinity Squared) Company in Scottsdale, Arizona — the same folks who make the Digest-a-Meal enzymes Ed will mention. (Their website is listed in Chapter 10.) The Lipochromizyme capsule contains lipase (the enzyme which digests fat), whose molecules are so microscopic that they can be absorbed directly into the body's bloodstream within 17 seconds of its ingestion. Just before each exercise session, I take one Lipochromizyme capsule, and it goes right to

work helping to convert fat to energy or replacing it with muscle. Muscle tissue burns calories even while at rest, and I have enough muscle tissue — even with the relatively small amount of exercise that I do — to enable me to eat as many calories as I want without significant weight gain, and to quickly lose weight when I cut back on calorie intake.

If there is any protein supplement powder in the house, I mix about two tablespoons of it into a half cup of water and drink it within forty-five minutes of the workout with the weights (when "worked" muscles are busy rebuilding themselves). Before bed, I also take the Digest-a-Meal digestive enzymes. With enzymes, nutrients in a balanced diet are so well absorbed, digested, and utilized that vitamin and mineral supplements probably become superfluous. I, however, take a few anyway, to be on the safe side. Just before bed I take vitamins C, E, a multiple, calcium/magnesium, and gingko biloba along with the Digest-a-Meal, with a large helping of water.

That's right! Lots of water just before bed. And I keep a quart of filtered water by my bedside. It's worth the inevitable trip to the rest room during the night because, along with the free radical damage, gradual dehydration is another factor in aging. Slow dehydration is widespread, but because it is so gradual, we do not recognize it. Each time we actually experience thirst, we are already severely dehydrated. Most of us do not drink enough water; also, the water we do drink has been treated with this and that, and the surface tension of the water molecules of "modern civilization" renders them more difficult for the cells of the body to absorb. The water lodges between cells, but is not easily absorbed through cell walls. Cells slowly lose more water than they replenish, and we gradually "shrivel."

Patrick Flanagan (creator of Microhydrin...Ed will mention it later) found that the key to the renowned longevity of the Hunza people was their drinking water, which originated from glaciers. The surface tension of that water (measured in units called "dynes") is less than ours; the water from the glacier is "wetter," more easily absorbed. Based upon extensive follow-up research, Dr. Flanagan developed Crystal Energy, a catalytic liquid which enhances the solvency of water. I recommend this product. Check it out at www.usvitamin.com/crystal-energy.

I make a goal of ingesting at least a half gallon of filtered water daily. There is a definite difference in my well-being since taking in more water.

Blessings

A game I play while running (I usually run in the early morning) is to look for at least one blessing. It can be a beautiful sunrise, a sliver of waning moon, a flock of honking geese, the beautiful showcased Handley High School building (so nicely lighted up before dawn), a pretty golden retriever, a friendly hello, the rain in my face... you get the idea. Running in the early morning provides the opportunity to see the seasons change as the rising sun moves up or down the eastern horizon, coming up earlier and earlier or later and later.

For me, the increase in metabolic activity while exercising can increase inspiration. I receive some of my best ideas and greatest "eureka!'s" when I am more "oxygenated." Ed will often count blessings while he runs. He thinks of a hundred things that he appreciates and counts them off. Blessings are everywhere; the more we look for them, the more we can think of, the more we see.

One of the most precious blessings that fitness after fifty can give us ladies is our men! On average, we women live longer than men, and can survive without them better than they can without us. Survive, yes. Thrive? No!! Won't it be wonderful when the nursing homes become empty, the doctor bills are minimal, and the older chicks (not biddies, but chicks!) all have a healthy husband or significant other or a large pool of choices of same, ready to boogie, travel, make love, play together with the grandchildren, read together in quiet companionship, hike, bike, walk a mile, golf, garden, get together with the other spring chickens over fifty, get together with the spring chickens under fifty, and... you fill in the rest.

Ed's postscript: *Three years ago I trained for months for the Apple Blossom Festival 10K, in hopes of finishing in the top five in my age group, achieving a 46-minute time, and receiving a trophy in just my second 10K race. One week before the race, I cajoled Mary into running the course during our regular Sunday run together. Then, having shown her that she could do it, I talked her into entering the race, itself — which she did. Here's the irony. She came in fifth in her age group and came away with a trophy and special recognition in the local paper (with virtually no training). I, on the other hand, having prepared well, came in eighth and received no trophy (even though I did reach my 46-minute goal). The last two years, Mary has come in second, garnering two more "trophies,"while I have finished sixth each year — just one place shy of being a medalist.*

This last summer, Mary was going to run with me in the Loudon- Street-Mile annual race. At the last minute, she pulled out due to the time constraints of her job. Bottom line, the winner in her age group was over two minutes slower than Mary's 10K (6-plus mile) pace. The winner was rewarded with a check for $75; Mary received half of that for a day's work as a docent at a local museum.

Mister Ed's Neighborhood

You have met the Masters of Fitness from around the nation; now, let's meet some who reside right here in my backyard. These "local" champions of fitness remind us that there are not just a handful of ultra-fit seniors scattered around the country, but rather, they are everywhere — some may be your neighbors. Multiply those in just my community times the thousands of communities nationwide and you get the picture. The sheer numbers show us that being fitter after 50 is within our grasp. I might add, these are mainly runners; we have hardly touched on the 50-plus skiers, martial artists, rock-climbers, etc. Imagine how many of these other Masters of Fitness there probably are.

One of the things I like about running is that it lends itself to comparisons of the running times of one person (often yourself) with the times of others and sets standards. This aspect of running allows us to measure our fitness level as well. Dr. Kenneth Cooper of the Cooper Aerobic Institute has devised a 12-minute test that correlates well with the testing performed in the laboratory to measure maximum oxygen uptake (MVO2) or cardiorespiratory fitness (also known as aerobic and endurance fitness). In Cooper's fitness lab, the subject walks/runs on a treadmill or rides a stationary bike while hooked up to state-of-the-art spirometric equipment to measure respiration and oxygen consumption. In the 12-minute cardiovascular test variation, the individual sees how many laps he can complete (running and/or walking) around a quarter-mile track in twelve minutes. Comparing the lab test results of thousands of clients with their track scores, Dr. Cooper and associates have established fairly reliable standards to measure one's aerobic fitness without the hassle of having to travel to his Dallas, Texas labs. We will use these standards to attest to the high fitness levels of our local Masters of Fitness. There are standards for men and women in 10-year age groupings (i.e., 20-29; 30-39; 40-49; and 50-59). To show that we can indeed be not just fit, but fitter after 50 than most 40, 30 or even 20-year-olds and to keep things simple, we will compare our local Masters with only the 20 to 29-year-old standards for excellence. I have taken the liberty to translate the laps-per-12-minutes scores into a one-mile average pace time for ease of comparison. The ratings are poor, fair, good, and excellent cardiorespiratory fitness. We need only zero in on the excellent standards for our purposes.

Excellent for men (20-29)
is a 7:16-mile pace for a little less than 1.75 miles.

Excellent for Women (20-29)
is an 8:53-mile pace for a little less than 1.38 miles.

As well as running/walking, there are also standards for swimming and cycling, too (see www.usarchery.org for complete age-graded charts).

To give you an idea of how fit our local Masters are, I recently ran a 3-mile race in 21 minutes and 12 seconds (a personal best). That comes out to 7:04 per mile or a 7:04-mile pace — which easily places me within the excellent range for 20 to 29-year-olds, and I am well past the half-century mark, as you well know by now. Now get this: *ALL* the individuals you are about to meet can beat me (and do on a regular basis) at this or some longer distance. Let's meet these runners whose dust I eat (or would if they would slow down enough for me to catch up to them).

229

Randy Wingfield, 56, is a member of the Shenandoah Valley Runners in the Northern Shenandoah Valley of Virginia, as are most of those that follow. He is an avid runner and a cyclist. A typical time for Randy in a 10K race is 42 minutes or less than seven minutes per mile for over six miles. Randy's times compared with the Cooper 12-minute test are well above excellent and would be in the elite level *for 20 to 29-year-olds* — if there were such a rating. Although Randy's personal bests (e.g., 34-minute 10Ks) came in his forties, he still can outrun most of the younger runners despite having had the cartilage surgically removed from his right knee as a young man, and the resulting arthritis. Randy says that the benefits of his running are "lower blood pressure, more energy, and needing only six hours of sleep."

Randy named Ray Kitchen and **Ray Gordon** as the fittest local Masters runners. He claims that, "Ray Gordon ran his age in the 440 [quarter mile] from age 55 to 75." That is, at age 55 he could run a quarter mile in 55 seconds or less; at 56 he was running the quarter in 56 seconds; and at 75, he could complete a lap around the track in 75 seconds. Keep in mind, the Olympic quarter-milers circle the track in about 45 seconds — so 55 seconds (and the other times) is quite impressive — and fast! Randy was also eager to share that Ray had set many track records including a world record for 60 to 64 year olds in the half mile with an astonishing 2:19 for the two lap race.

Ray was the founder of Shenandoah Valley Runners in the mid 1970's, and at 83 twice came "running" in from chopping wood to answer my telephone calls and verify that he had indeed run his age in the quarter mile for 21 straight years and set a world record in the half mile for 60 year olds.

In his mid-thirties, **Ray Kitchen** was jogging a mile or two a couple times a week. At age 40, to lose weight and get his high blood pressure under control, he decided to get serious about his running, and boy, did he ever! For the next nine years he kept setting new personal bests until by age 49, he was running 38 to 39-minute 10K's — that is a blistering 6:30/mile pace. Ray also set longterm goals to:

1. Run a marathon
2. Qualify for and run in the Boston Marathon
3. Complete a 50-miler

Ray achieved them all and then some. He has not only run a marathon — he has run Boston nine times. His 50-miler turned into 10 consecutive JFK 50-Mile Races — all but one of them in under ten hours (with a personal best of 8:30).

Why does Ray run? He runs and races because he enjoys running, loves the challenge of competing, likes the feeling of accomplishment, and reaps many health benefits. For example, at work a couple of years ago, the employees were given a MVO2 breathing test. While the results of the test showed that Ray had the lungs of a 40 year old, a co-worker of a similar age was informed that he had the lungs of a 70 year old.

Ray, a football player (not a runner) in high school, says that the secret to his success "is training." His advice to us is to remember that "the biggest thing you can do is [to] set goals."

The first thing I noticed about **Burr Grim** was that his legs end at his armpits; Burr was built to run, and has he ever. He was in the top echelon of U.S. runners in his youth — racing the world's best runners (e.g., Jim Beatty and Ron Dulaney) in his heyday. Now 68, he is still going strong, while most of his world-class competitors have long since traded in their running shoes for a middle-age spread.

I interviewed Burr at a local 3-mile race. He told me about going to the Senior Olympics at William and Mary College, when he was just a youngster of sixty, and winning four gold medals. He entered races varying in length from the one mile to the 10K. One of his proudest moments was at this competition when he lapped all the other runners in a 4-lap one-mile race (all or most of whom were in their fifties and as much as 10 years younger then he). In all, he took part in four Senior Olympics, garnering a total of about 18 gold medals. Another cherished accomplishment that he shared with me was his 3:08 run at the Marine Corps Marathon, also when he was sixty. This despite the fact that he ran the second half of the marathon with an injured leg.

As we warmed up before the 3-miler, Burr told me that he "had worked all night doing heavy lifting" in his factory job. He added that he "had just got off work" and on top of this he was "not in racing shape." As the race started, there right in front of me, among a couple hundred racers, was Burr. "Too bad he was worn out from working all night, out of shape, and twelve years older than I," I thought. "I'll just fall in right behind him and then pass him near the end of the race." Well, a funny thing happened on the way to the finish line. Although he didn't look like he was putting forth that much effort, he kept getting further and further in front of me until he — well, he disappeared. Though I ran my fastest 3-mile time ever, when I reached the finish line, he had long since finished and wandered off to probably do some push-ups or something. Too bad he was so tired; otherwise, I could have really given him a run for his money — or not!

Burr's fitness activities include running, swimming, and a physically demanding job. Staying strong, a good diet, and peace of mind are his secret weapons. His advice for us, "You have to stay strong — physically strong." Burr's final bit of wisdom for us, "If you want to do what I do, you'll have to think like I think!"

As with Burr, **Jason Page**'s running career started with high school track and field. As a young adult he was a very successful runner, as shown by his National Junior Postal 10-Mile Championship in 1964. Instead of retiring from running, he has continued to run because he enjoys it and for the health benefits. At 57, he still runs a 39-minute 10K. His recent 19:59 for a hilly 5K race comes out to a 6:26/mile pace — well below the 7:16 needed to be in excellent shape (as a 20-year-old) according to the Cooper 12-minute test (which, by the way, is run on a flat track — not a 5K course with hills to negotiate). Any way you cut it, Jason is definitely fitter after 50 (as proven by the fact that his cardiovascular fitness score is better than even a 20-year-old who is "officially" proclaimed to be in excellent shape).

Unlike Burr Grim, it was his wheels, not his legs, that I noticed first when I met runner, **Chuck Raper.** He had driven to the 3-miler in his sweats and an elegant white stretch limousine. Obviously, he has a unique way of stretching before a race. But his car is not what we are interested in here. Right? RIGHT?

At age 58, Chuck runs 10K's at a 6:40 per mile pace and marathons at a 7:56-mile clip. Compared with our 12-minute test standards, these are remarkable times for *any age.* However, Chuck wasn't always this fit. When he started running in 1982, he was 5 foot 9 inches tall (still is), weighed 205 pounds (not any more), and got winded just walking up a flight of stairs. Now he is 155 pounds, with an excellent body-fat percentage of 13.9 (15 is ideal — 23 is average for men) and is a superb athlete who, besides running, swims and bikes.

Why did Chuck change all those years ago? He didn't like the way he looked and felt and "wanted to get into good shape." Why does he continue to run and race nearly 20 years later? He perseveres, he says, "To maintain fitness and not [have to] watch every calorie or the fat content [of foods]." He also likes the health benefits, fun of racing, and the camaraderie. Chuck's advice for us, don't just start exercising — for best results make a commitment to a total change in lifestyle and make it forever. Finally, don't exclude foods from your diet (i.e., don't deprive yourself), but always be disciplined in your eating.

We have heard from the men. Now it is time to get the female perspective.

As with Chuck, **Sandy Adams** took stock of her fitness around age forty and didn't like what she saw. Specifically, she found that due to her sedentary lifestyle, which included a desk job, she was "in terrible shape!" As Sandy puts it, "Back then, a couple of flights of steps and I was out of breath. When I began walking with some friends, after two blocks we were tired and wanted to turn around and go back."

That was then; this is now. Recently Sandy set an age-group record for 50-54-year-old women with a 41-minute 10K at Pikes Peak, Maryland. That is better than a 7-minute per mile pace for just over six miles; if you recall, the 12-minute endurance test for 20-year-old women rates as excellent an 8:53-mile pace (for less than a mile and a half). That places Sandy off the charts, in the stratosphere, somewhere between awesome and "holy cow." This 52-year-old mother of one also runs in the 3:20's for the marathon (about 7:45/mile) and has a 50-miler to her credit. Sandy continues to run, she says, "for the health benefits, weight control (it obviously works) and the people she meets."

As awesome as Sandy is, she is in awe of her friend, the very athletic **Kathy Smart.** This is partly because Kathy is a multi-sport talent — not just a runner. Kathy, at 59, still enjoys biking, swimming, kayaking, lifting weights, triathlons, 50-mile trail-running races, marathons and who knows what else. Why would someone almost 60 years old want to continually stretch her limits? For enjoyment, of course, but also, she says, "to keep my weight down, stay healthy and because I like to compete." Like most of the others, one of her motivators is the camaraderie she enjoys during training and at competitions.

Where does Kathy get the energy and strength to be the human version of a perpetual-motion machine? First and foremost, she obviously loves these sporting activities and events. Beyond that, she has a few aces up her sleeve. For one, she cross-trains to save wear and tear on her body/joints (avert repetitive-motion injuries) and to alleviate the boredom of doing the same activities day after day. Kathy runs 4 or 5 days a week, mostly on trails and dirt roads, for distances of 5 to 15 miles. She puts in somewhere between 25 and 35 miles a week except when getting ready for a 35k or 50k when her weekly mileage may go up to 40 or 45 miles. She bikes twice a week between March and November, but has eliminated swimming from her training regimen since she moved away from the local municipal pool. Twice a week she takes a 90-minute yoga class and she stretches each morning for 15 to 30 minutes. She finds the yoga and stretching very helpful in keeping her moving as she ages. Two days a week she lifts weights (the importance of which too many runners overlook).

As far as fuel is concerned, she loads up on fruits and vegetables (sound familiar?) and limits desserts. She supplements with vitamins C and E, calcium, a muli-vitamin, and glucosamine. She believes firmly that the glucosamine is a big help in keeping her joints from getting stiff from all her activities. The only sports-related potion she uses is GU (like a gooey Gatorade). During long training runs and races she consumes some GU every 45 minutes to keep her blood-sugar level even (no bonking for Kathy). Kathy's advice for us is to start out slowly, join a gym, and get help in the form of a personal trainer or mentor.

You will not find our final lady running in a road race or lifting weights at the gym. **Pat Rice** travels in other circles — the martial arts in general and Qigong and Tai Chi in particular. Pat has trained privately with well-known Masters of Taijiquan (Tai Chi) in China. She must have been an "A" student, because in 1986 and 1987 she placed first in

Taijiquan and first in Push-Hands at the U.S. National Kung-Fu/Wushu Competitions in Houston, Texas. More recently, in 1999, she was named one of the 100 Most Influential Persons In Martial Arts in the U.S. in the past 100 years by *Inside Kung Fu* magazine. You may have heard of some of her co-honorees: Bruce Lee, David Carradine, Jackie Chan, Jean-Claude Van Damme, Chuck Norris, Kareem Abdul Jabbar, Billy Blanks, and Jhoon Rhee. An additional honor, bestowed on her in 2001, was her induction into *Inside Kung Fu's* Hall of Fame.

So what is Tai Chi? According to Pat, "Tai Chi is practiced as a series of movements, connected in a flowing pattern, and governed by principles of correct body usage." It has been developed over thousands of years as a martial art, an exercise, and a moving meditation. It is practiced as slow, precise movements and is said to help with stress relief, strength, balance, flexibility, improved posture, and cardiovascular endurance.

Let's listen to Pat as she describes her Tai Chi sessions and helps us understand what exactly Tai Chi is and what it can do for us:

I practice a set routine of tai chi that takes about 20-25 minutes. During this time, my focus is on establishing and maintaining a mind-body connection. This means that I put my concentration onto what I am doing, being totally "in the moment" so that I am conscious of the movements and their effects in various areas of my body. I check certain areas, such as shoulders and lower back, and deliberately release tension from those muscles as I move. I also need to be aware of keeping proper alignment through the entire body. The movements are guided by long-established principles that aid the physical and mental processes. Some of the effects of these sub-activities are heightened ability to focus the mind for extended periods of time, strengthening muscles in the arms and legs, extended stamina, better balance, and general relief of both physical and mental stress.

As for qigong, Pat says:

"Qigong" means "energy work" and it's a method of working with the natural energies of the body to enhance health. For example, breathing patterns and physical movements and meditations are among these methods. I also do some qigong on a daily basis. Qigong and tai chi have many

235

elements in common, and I believe that the practice of both art forms gives me the health and stamina that I have at my age.

Does it really work? After all, we Americans tend to cling to the no-pain, no-gain mentality, such as is found in road racing; and this art form is anything but a race. Pat tells about one Art Perkins who was involved in an automobile accident that caused both severe body and traumatic brain injury. After many months of physical therapy, he was released because there was nothing more "they" could do for him. For thirty years he had an unsteady gait and walked with a cane. Then, after just three years at Pat's martial arts studio, he came to Tai Chi class one day without his cane. Tai Chi had completed what physical therapy had started, and helped him overcome over 30 years of poor balance, lack of strength, and general coordination problems.

Pat also told about a 102-year-old Tai Chi Master she met in Beijing, China. Each day he would traverse six flights of stairs, coming and going (climbing and descending) to perform his daily Tai Chi movements in the park. This Master/teacher walked independently (no cane, walking stick, etc.), gracefully, and took no medications. He, likewise, is an example of what Tai Chi can do for us.

What proof do we have that Pat is fitter than the average 20 or 30-year-old? With runners, we can use their race times to see how they compare with others, and set standards. But how do we measure the non-competitive athlete for fitness? First, when you look at this 59-year-old, you won't see any sign of middle-age spread or stress-producing postures, so prevalent in Americans over the age of forty. Pat impresses you with her lithe figure, quiet confidence, and her grace. She takes no medication, has boundless energy (efficiently used), and has not had the flu or other maladies for years and years. Pat balances her Tai Chi and Qigong with long, enjoyable walks and hikes.

Pat wants us to know that one can start Tai Chi at any age, no matter how out-of-shape he or she has become. It is the perfect activity to reestablish calm and self-assuredness in anyone's stress-filled, hectic lifestyle. Pat says, "Get started — don't wait!"

Mary and Ed's Fix of Supplements

Now let's turn our attention to some dietary supplements that Mary and I have found helpful in our ascent to being fitter after 50. Like our senior fitness champs, we have found that the secret to getting fitter after 50 lies mainly in our diet, exercise and mindset, and not with supplements. There are very healthy, fit and long-lived individuals scattered around the world who have never heard of, never mind dabbled in, CoQ10 or ginseng, Korean, American or otherwise. That having been said, here are our favorite supplements.

Protein Powder

In one study, sedentary men and women and highly-trained athletes were fed diets of 2.4 grams of protein per kilogram of body weight and then .86 grams of protein per kilogram. After about two weeks, it was found that they had gained weight/muscle no faster on the 2.4 gram diet than on the .86 gram version. In another study, beginning body-builders gained no more muscle and strength on 2.6 grams of protein/kg feedings than they did on a 1.4 gram/kg diet.

The secret to gaining bulk/muscle is to eat more calories (from nutritious foods, including high protein sources) and to perform intense strength-building workouts. When one does that, he can't help but get the 120 to 180 grams of protein recommended for a 200-pound athlete. During the Body For Life Challenge, I gained about ten pounds of muscle, but I don't know whether it was as a result of the added protein powder, the six meals a day, the intense-strength workouts, or a combination of all three. I have a hunch that it was the meals and workouts, because I've downed a lot of protein shakes since then without gaining much more muscle at all. Not only hasn't my body bulked up, but my wallet has gotten skinnier in the process. I do believe that we can get all the protein we need to be fitter after 50 from a healthful, well-planned diet of everyday foods. But I still enjoy the convenience, protein "insurance" and taste of my fruit (strawberry, blueberry, red raspberry, ...) smoothie protein shakes.

Creatine

One supplement that that I have found very beneficial is creatine monohydrate. Creatine is an amino acid (the chief component of protein) that is found primarily in the muscles of the body. Although it can be obtained by eating beef, salmon and other creatures (about two grams/one pound of meat), one would have to eat an unhealthy amount of roasted beast to get the recommended 5 grams per day for fitness gains. I don't aspire to eat that much fish or meat, so I supplement with the pure creatine powder from time to time. It helps maintain the availability of energy during intense workouts, such as weightlifting and sprints. It can also aid in the recovery time needed between bouts of intense exercise. About 250 creatine studies have been conducted and 95 percent of them show an increase in exercise capacity. The use of creatine in concert with quality training can lead to 5 to 15 percent increases in strength. I have personally noticed a definite difference when using it.

Antioxidants and Microhydrin

When foods and other compounds in our body are oxidized, they lose a hydrogen electron, which makes them free radicals. These free radicals, in an effort to find balance, steal electrons from the cells of our tissues and organs. It is this cellular damage which is at the root of biological "aging." Antioxidants such as the familiar vitamins C and E and beta-carotene, give up an electron to neutralize the free radicals and make them harmless. In doing so, however, they themselves then become free radicals, but weaker, less-destructive versions.

In recent years, scientist and visionary Patrick Flanagan discovered the existence of a hydrogen atom in glaciers, fresh fruits, raw vegetables, and raw meat that has not one electron, but two. This negatively-charged hydrogen anion easily gives up its second loosely-bound electron. Through years of research, Flanagan found a way to attach this hydrogen anion to food-grade silica, forming a powder which he has found to have the antioxidant power of 10,000 glasses of fresh-squeezed orange juice. It retails under the name Microhydrin and it is the only antioxidant that doesn't become a free radical itself when it neutralizes free radicals, because what is left (the byproduct) is pure hydrogen, which then combines with oxygen molecules to form water, which the body can use.

For more information about this amazing anti-aging supplement, go to www.rbcnow.com or call (972)893-4000.

Even if we use Microhydrin (I do — have for years off and on), we still need our other antioxidants with their cascading neutralizing effect on one another, and I get my beta-carotene, "C" and "E" and myriad other antioxidants mostly from healthful foods. I'm looking at a study on vitamin C reported by Joseph A. Vita, M.D., associate professor of medicine at Boston University's School of Medicine in [where else?] Boston, Massachusetts. It says that a study of 26 individuals with severely-blocked arteries discovered that high doses of vitamin C helped their arteries open normally within two hours. These researchers theorize that the "C" works by suppressing superoxide, a substance that interferes with the body's natural means of opening arteries. Blocked arteries cause limited blood flow to the heart, causing angina and heart attacks. If this study is corroborated by future research and found to be the real deal, how fantastic would that be? Instead of risky and costly by-pass surgery, we'd be able to take a vitamin pill. Antioxidants, whether they be the common vitamins C and E, the newly-created Microhydrin, or some as-yet-undiscovered miracle worker, can be appreciated and harnessed for our highest good.

A little footnote here is in order. A couple of years ago, I had a large brown or dark spot in my left eye's visual field which was interferring with my vision. I have one farsighted eye and one that is nearsighted. This "spot" was in the nearsighted eye. It got to the point where I had trouble seeing to shave and couldn't read any more except under very bright lighting. I especially had difficulty with reading the newspaper. I treated my condition by consuming two generous helpings of cooked carrots and two to four Microhydrin capsules each day for about a month. Lo! and behold, the "spot" gradually diminished until it disappeared altogether, never to return. Thank you, antioxidants and other nutrients!

Digestive Enzymes
There was a time a few years ago when I couldn't do chin-ups or even straighten my arms when hanging from a chinning bar. This painful condition in my shoulder joints lasted for about a year. Live blood analysis of a drop of my blood, using

the darkfield microscope technology, showed my blood to be a mess. Some of the crystalline (or calcified) material floating around in my blood was said to be the culprit causing my problem, as it was probably being deposited in my joints. At the time, I had just been introduced to digestive enzymes. The microscopic size of these particular enzymes allowed them to be transported directly into the blood stream, bypassing the digestive process, and as I watched the TV monitor, I witnessed first hand the enzymes disintegrating the crystalline troublemakers. To make a long story short, after about a month of loading up on this enzyme product, Digest-A-Meal, the pain in my shoulders disappeared. Whether this was the result of the placebo effect or an actual medical/nutritional intervention, I don't know. What I do know is that I took this product (with no other significant lifestyle changes) and my pain went away. Not very scientific, but I'll take it. For more information, check out www.infinity2.com.

In summary, I (Ed) use creatine because it helps with my strength workouts. The other product I take is the super-antioxidant, Microhydrin. It gives me pleasure to think that the Microhydrin is busy for hours every day scavenging for free radicals and rendering them impotent.

Besides these dietary supplements, there are some gadgets that I've enjoyed using in my quest to be fitter after 50. In my hope that at least one of them will be of some assistance to you, here they are.

VitaMix Super 5000

The VitaMix is like a blender, but better; it's like a juicer, but better. If you are like me, you don't always feel like eating an apple or chewing on a stalk of celery, but you do want the nourishment, the youth-producing benefits, of five to twelve fruits and vegetables a day.

The VitaMix is so easy to use. Just cut up and throw the whole apple or other produce into the VitaMix with some water (no need to peel or core the apple, just wash it first). The VitaMix quickly (in mere seconds) grinds — pulverizes — the fruit and/or vegetable (in most cases skin, seeds and all) into a nutritious and delicious drink. It does not throw out the pulp (containing about half the vitamins, minerals and other nutrients and most of the fiber) like juicers do. We get all the nutrients and fiber of the whole fruit or vegetable, but in microscopic-sized particles that are more easily absorbed by our digestive system. Also, the clean-up is much easier and quicker than with a juicer, or even a blender.

On the downside, it's a very noisy machine and more expensive than most juicers and blenders, but as you can see, it is worth it! Call 1-800-848-2649 for details or go to www.vitamix.com.

Freeze-Framer

The Freeze-Framer is a simple and fun-to-use software/hardware program for your computer. By placing a finger on a sensor, one's heart rhythms are displayed on the monitor. The significance of the heart's signals is that the heart's magnetic field is more than 5,000 times stronger than the brain's; the amplitude of its electrical field is 60 times greater. These powerful signals from the heart are transmitted to every cell of the body *and beyond* and all the other systems of the body entrain to the heart. By merely changing one's thoughts/feelings and focusing on the heart region, one finds his heart-rate-variability pattern changing from incoherent (catabolic) to coherent (anabolic); from a stressful, aging signal to an invigorating, life-enhancing one. Using this biofeedback-like instrument, we can quickly master two stress-reduction techniques that can be used almost anywhere and any time to help us become fitter after 50. This is a life-transforming tool of the Institute of HeartMath — one of the "Eight That Work."

Heart-Rate Monitors

The kind of heart-rate monitor I recommend is one that is comprised of a transmitter held to the chest by an elastic band and a receiver that attaches to the wrist like a wrist watch. A HRM can be used while walking, biking, running, etc. to let us know if we are overstressing our system or not challenging ourselves enough. This is usually done by setting a heart-rate range or training range (e.g., 110 bpm to 130 bpm) within which we wish to stay during our exercise session or during a portion of it. The better models of watches will alert us by visual and/or auditory signal when our heart rate deviates from our intended range. Dr. Philip Maffetone (one of the "Eight That Work") relies heavily on heart rate monitors to train athletes from novice to professional. In his writings, he explains how to determine one's optimal training range for burning fat/aerobic workouts. I might mention here that in one study, runners who used HRM's to set their pace lost more weight than those who took their pulse manually.

Although it is not essential gear, the HRM is much more convenient and accurate (once it is set — see your local rocket scientist for assistance) than frequently stopping and manually taking a pulse. A dependable brand is Polar and a good HRM can run from 100 to 200 dollars. I love mine!

The Sports Breather

This pocket-sized device is "weight training" for the respiratory muscles. It increases lung capacity and greatly improves circulation for more life-giving oxygen to the body. Use it while at stoplights, watching TV, or surfing the web to get a workout for your respiratory system without leaving your chair. But don't let any teenagers catch you puffing and blowing on it, as they might just break a rib laughing at you. I used this device successfully to train for my only 10-miler and by my good results, I do believe it helped. If you have respiratory shortcomings, check with your doctor, as this might (or might not be) "just what the doctor ordered." For more information, call (877) 419-1729 or check out www.j-f-financial.com/sportsbreather.

Total Gym

If you are looking for a reasonably priced, quality home gym, you need look no further than the Total Gym. There are several models from which to choose and dozens of different exercises can be performed on these gravity-based machines. You lie on a sled which moves up and down a variable incline as you push and pull on various handles and gadgets. The level of resistance, a percentage of your body weight, coincides with the angle of the incline. The base model sells for around $200. I've found mine a very convenient, effective strength builder.

Athletic Shoes

The right shoes can make all the difference. I have athletic shoes that I would never use for running and others that are made for running. Uncomfortable or inappropriate shoes can dampen one's enthusiasm for working out, or even cause injury. In her 23 injury-free years of running, Helen Klein suffered through just a single week of leg pain (iliotibial band friction syndrome) when her shoe sponsor "improved" the stability and support of her shoe.

We don't need the most expensive shoes, but neither do we want cheap ones. Athletic shoe reviews/guides in sports and consumer magazines often find that the mid-range-priced shoes outperform the most expensive models (e.g., for years Helen used a mid-range, $59 shoe). Such reviews can help us narrow down our choices and find the best footwear for our sport's needs. We can also check with knowledgeable hikers, bikers or runners for their suggestions.

What Do We Really Need

In the end, our Masters of Fitness would have us know that magical potions and miracle-promising equipment do not a fit person make. It all goes back to desire and belief. If our "why" is strong enough, the "how" (and the equipment/supplements necessary) will come. Think more often about what you desire and *dwell* upon why you want it. Train and dream commensurate to your goals so that you can really believe you can achieve them, and you will.

Your Story

We have heard Ed and Mary's stories and the stories from Mr. Ed's Neighborhood. Dozens of Masters of Fitness have been met and their secrets learned. Now it's your turn.

Remember the story of the prodigal son in the Bible (Luke 15:11)? The younger brother strayed and wasted his wealth on riotous living, while the older sibling stayed with the father and served him well. Yet, when the transgressor returned home, his father accepted him with open arms and gifts even more lavish than those he had bestowed upon the ever-faithful son.

So it is with us. We can spend our health recklessly and squander it over the years until we are in dismal shape. Yet, when we return home — get fit and healthy — it is as if we had never left our fitness behind. We are lavished with the rich rewards of being fit no matter how recent the conversion and irrespective of how late in life we return.

Imagine what it would mean to you and yours for you to be fitter after 50!

CHAPTER 10 FITTER AFTER 50'S TOP 40

In this era of information overkill, what is important is not how many gigabites of RAM or factoids we can lug around inside our heads, but rather that we know how (read that, where) to access specific bits of knowledge on how to be fitter after 50, etc. when we have occasion for it. Next to my bed is a teetering stack of books and magazines, chock full of fascinating bits of information, which threatens to topple during the night and bury me alive — luckily I am fit enough to dig my way out. To avoid this peril, not to mention the clutter, you may want to rely more on the computer for storage and retrieval of information.

Here are web sites that I have found useful or interesting. If you have not yet veered onto the information highway, then you can go to your local library for access and help; you can even print out the data/articles onto good, old reliable paper to read and study later at your leisure. I do not endorse any of these dot-coms as the mother lode of right answers. Some I know well and use, and others I just know of. In other words, be a smart and wary consumer. Checking in at number 40 is:

#40 AARP.org/Wellness
American Association of Retired Person's wellness page * Wellness newsletter * Featured articles * Staying fit * Eating well * Managing stress * Aging well

#39 RunInjuryFree.com
"Running Injury Free with Jeff Galloway" * Galloway Gear * Promina Corporate Challenge * Pace groups * Newsletter * Nutrition * Training * Ask Jeff

#38 MacroBiotics.org
Macrobiotics Online: a natural, holistic approach to health * Macrobiotic diet * Macrobiotic lifestyle * Case histories * Articles * Recipes * Catalog of organic whole foods, cookware and books

#37 LEF.org
Life Extension Foundation * Reversing aging * Life Extension daily news * Search LE magazine back issues

#36 FitnessLink.com
"Reshape Your World" * Reshape your: body — mind — diet — career * Men's locker room * Women's locker room * The juice bar

#35 StrengthCoach.com
Personalized training program for a specific sport (for the serious athlete) * Meet your performance potential * Nutrition * Research * Games to play online

#34 RideFast.com
Carmichael Training Systems by Chris Carmichael (3-time Tour de France Champion Lance Armstrong's coach) * World-class coaching via the web for cycling, running and other sports * $79/month to $499/month — minimum 4 to 6 months

#33 WeightWatchers.com
Success stories * Delicious recipes * Fitness * Today's focus * Assess yourself * Community * Recipe swap * Quizzes * Find a meeting

#32 CoolRunning.com
Running race event locator * Entry forms * Posted results * Running news * Pace calculator

#31 Womens-Running.com
Women's running from Runner's World * Getting started * Body * Self * Women's concerns * Women's writes * Women's weekly * Ask the athlete * My training diary * Community

#30 JorgeCruise.com
Named #1 Online Fitness trainer by Yahoo! * Weight Loss For Busy People * 8 Minutes in the Morning (book) * Testimonials * Shopping * $10,000 8-Minute Challenge * Ask Jorge your question

#29 USMS.org
United States Masters Swimming * Swimming for life for all ages (19 to over 100) * Fitness * Training * Competition * Fun * Merchandise * Swimming links

#28 MensHealth.com
The Men's Health Challenge * Mens Health Personal Trainer: Customized programs with animated exercise demonstrations * Daily tips * Contests * Surveys * Ask the girl next door * News * Talk to us * Fitness * Sex * Weight loss * Health

#27 Obesity.Chair.ULaval.ca/index.htm
Research from Laval University in Quebec, Canada * Prevalence, causes and consequences of obesity * Group support * Behavioral therapy * Diet and nutrition * Weight management

#26 AHealthyMe.com
A healthy approach to fitness, family and fun * Ask Dr. Anne * In the news * Senior health * Lifestyle and wellness * Fitness and nutrition * Medical library * Cool tools

#25 RealAge.com
Health tools and tips for living Younger * Real Age test * Tip of the day * Real Age diet * Health news * Healthy Bytes (personalized health and lifestyle newsletter)

#24 RunnersWorld.com
Runner's World magazine web site * Beginner's program * Shoes and gear reviews * Training & racing * Race & marathon calendar * News references * Records & stats * Highlights of current RW magazine * Masters' world & national records (in 5-year groupings from 40 to 94)

#23 SitAndBeFit.com
A wide variety of award-winning videos for seniors with limiting conditions, such as arthritis and heart disease * Exercise equipment * Articles * Videos in $20 range * Nonprofit

#22 DrMcDougall.com
McDougall Wellness Center — One of Eight that Work *
McDougall programs * Effects of nutrition on disease *
McDougall products * Holiday recipes * Total Health Solution
video program

#21 NewRunner.com
Step-by-step guide for new runners * Quote of the week *
Motivate Me! * Secrets of my success: Oprah Winfrey * Training
log * 10 great reasons to run * A Runner's World magazine site

#20 Canoe.ca
A Canadian site — click on C-Health for a wealth of info.:
Fitness * Nutrition * Eating scorecard * A list of Canadian
health-related associations and foundations * Alternative
health dictionary

#19 Chopra.com
Mind-Body Medicine's Deepak Chopra, M.D.'s site * Ask
Deepak * Quote of the day * Spiritual law of the day * Recipe
of the week * Excerpts from Deepak's teachings * Calendar of
events * Reversal of aging

#18 Women.com
Everything a lady would want to know and then some —
click on Fitness, Health & Fitness, or Food * Workout
personality quiz * Weight quiz * Healthy eater quiz * Daily
meal planner * Walking calculator * Workout planner * Organic
produce * Recipe finder

#17 Barnett-Fitness.com
The award-winning Barnett Training System * Bodybuilding
* Nutrition * Aerobics * Flexibility * Workbook * Video *
Consultations

#16 TNP.com
The Natural Pharmacist * Look up condition, herb,
supplement, drug or therapy * See how natural treatment
compares to conventional medicine * Science based

#15 MedlinePlus.gov
A service of the National Library of Medicine/National Institutes of Health * Health topics * Information on conditions, diseases and wellness

#14 HalHigdon.com
Training programs for beginning, intermediate, and advanced runners: * 5Ks * 8Ks *10Ks * 15Ks * 10-milers * Half-marathons * Marathons * Ultra-marathons * Also, skiing, art, travel and more

#13 Compuserve.com/health/
Health E Tools: Find a doctor * Health risk appraisal * Diet & fitness journal (track calories & exercise) * *Health Calculator:* Body mass index * Healthy weight * Waist-to-hip ratio * Daily requirements for calories, carbohydrates, fat (minimum to maximum), protein, and calcium * Target heart rate range * Calories burned/minute in a chosen fitness activity * *Exercise Match* — Find an activity that fits your personality and lifestyle

#12 NutrActive.com
Weight loss center * *Fitness Center:* Personalized fitness programs & supplements * Cooking and diabetes centers * Book & video store

#11 Abraham-Hicks.com
Audio tapes, online transcripts and workshops on the Science of Deliberate Creation and the Art of Allowing our *well*-being * Find out how we create health and sickness and can become fitter after 50

#10 HeartMath.com
Study the research behind the HeartMath stress-reduction techniques (one of the Eight that Work) * Source for ordering books, music CDs, Freeze-Framers, and other products to produce coherent, vitality-producing heart rhythms * Workshops & seminars

#9 ChooseToMove.org
An American Heart Association/Cooper Aerobic Institute site * A fun, free and flexible 12-week aerobic program for women * Gradually work up to 30 minutes per day of exercise * Healthy eating * Weight management

#8 Workout.com
Exercise Zone: Over 500 exercises in 9 categories * *Program Zone:* Increased muscle size * Sports training * Weight loss/decrease body fat * Cardio-endurance * In home/traveler * Rehabilitation * Muscle toning/definition * Over 1,000 professionally-designed programs * *Diet Zone:* Lose 10 pounds by ___ (personalized)

#7 ACEfitness.org
Site of the nonprofit American Council on Exercise * Become a certified personal trainer * Find an ACE-certified personal trainer, fitness instructor or health club in your locale * Health E-tips Newsletter * Fitness Matters magazine (former-tree-and-magazine-rack-type) * ACE Fit Facts

#6 Nutri-Facts.com
Source for nutrition facts on about 6,000 foods & drinks (protein, fat, sugar, fiber, vitamins & mineral content) * Body mass index calculator * Calories-burning calculator * Calorie intake calculator

#5 NetFit.co.uk/netfit.htm
An online fitness club run by some of the United kingdom's top personal trainers * Fitness tests with charts to find fitness level * 200 fitness exercises/programs demonstrated & explained * Fitness tips * Design your own program

#4 About.com
Information on everything under the sun — scroll down to fitness/wellness * Walk of Life (free 10-week program) * Cool Running 9-week training program (to run first 5K or 5 miler) * Senior health * Avon 3-day walks (60 miles to annihilate breast cancer) * Low-fat cooking * Start a cycling program * Alternative medicine * Age-graded tables (how your racing time compares with that of a 20 or 30-year-old)

#3 BodyForLife.com

One of the Eight That Work * Personalized strength training program * Find your VO2 max * Find your bodyfat percentage * Find your target heart rate * Real video/instructions for strength exercises * Recipes & menus * Nutrition guidelines * Million Dollar Body For Life Challenge

#2 ThriveOnLine.com

Webby Awards winner 2000 — best health site * Lifestyle assessment * Park & trail guide * Fitness planner (free, personalized workout) * Medical library * Parent company, Oxygen Media, "aims to present the world through women's eyes"

#1 StrongWomen.com

One of the Eight That Work * Choose from 3 strength-building programs: Vibrant Aging - Stay Slim - Strong Bones (general programs — free & personalized programs — $29.95/6 months) * Animated exercise illustrations * E-newsletter * Archival issues * Recipes * Printable exercise log * Order "Strong Women ..." books

Information Please

Here are some more websites, plus the top 40, organized by categories for your convenience. Many of these sites could be placed in more than one category, but I placed them where I felt they belonged by priority. Have fun navigating this sea of knowledge.

Wellness/Health

WebMD.com *** DrWhitaker.com *** CDC.gov/nccdphp/dnpa/npa-proj.htm *** AmericanGeriatrics.org *** ThirdAge.com *** NLM.NIH.gov (United States National Library of Medicine) *** HealthFinder.gov *** InfoAging.org *** CBSHealthWatch.Medscape.com *** ncbi.nlm.nih.gov/pubmed/ *** PubMedCentral.nih.gov/ *** ahrg.gov/ppip/50plus/ *** HealthScout.com *** HealthLetter.Tufts.edu *** hnrc.Tufts.edu/ *** KeiserInstituteOnAging.com *** iVillageHealth.com *** Health.Discovery.com *** RDHealth.com *** HealthyAging.net/campaign.htm ***AARP.org/wellness (40)

*** LEF.org (Life Extension Foundation - 37) *** Self.com *** MensHealth.com (28) *** AHealthyMe.com (26) *** RealAge.com (25) *** Canoe.ca (click on C-Health - 20) *** Women.com (click on fitness, health, wellness or food - 18) *** MedlinePlus.gov (15) *** CompuServe.com/health/ (13) *** ThriveOnLine.com (2)

General Fitness
SeniorFitness.net *** FloridaFitness.com *** FitnessOnLine.com *** SeniorJournal.com *** Aworkout.com *** 50Plus.org *** HumanKinetics.com *** JustMove.org *** FitnessLink.com (36) *** Obesity.Chair.ULaval.ca/index.htm (27) *** SitAndBeFit.com (23) *** NutrActive.com (12) *** ChooseToMove.org (9) *** Workout.com (8) *** ACEfitness.org (7) *** NetFit.co.uk/netfit.htm (5) *** VO2MaxUSA.com *** JorgeCruise.com (30) *** HowToStretch.com

Diet/Nutrition
MuscleMaster.com *** eDiets.com *** 5Aday.com *** AboutProduce.com *** GSSIWeb.com (Gatorade Sports Science Institute) *** RecipeFinder.com *** cspiNet.org (Nutrition Action Health Letter) *** CalorieControl.org *** EatRight.org *** CyberDiet.com *** FightFatAfter40.com *** Macrobiotics.org (38) *** DrMcDougall.com (22) *** Nutri-Facts.com (6) *** GlycemicIndex.com

Strength Training
EAS.com *** MuscleMedia.com *** CyberPump.com *** BodyBuilding.com *** NaturalBodyBuilding.com *** StrengthCoach.com (35) *** Barnett-Fitness.com (17) *** BodyForLife.com (3) *** StrongWomen.com (1)

Running
MastersTrack.com *** MarathonAndBeyond.com *** RunThePlanet.com *** MarathonMan.org (Jerry Dunn's site) *** WhereToRun.com *** MarathonGuide.com *** OD100.org (Old Dominion 100 Miler) *** RunningInjuryFree.com (39) *** CoolRunning.com (32) *** Womens-Running.com (31) *** RunnersWorld.com (24) *** NewRunner.com (21) *** HalHigdon.com (14) *** RunnersWeb.com

Other Sports
SwimGold.org *** SurfingForLife.com *** Triathlete.com ***
OutsideMag.com/bodywork *** Nexternal.com (Tai Chi, yoga,
Qigong, & martial arts) *** EasyTaiChi.com ***
WalkingMag.com *** RideFast.com (34) *** USMS.org (masters
swimming - 29) *** Trails.com

Mind-Body
DreamLife.com *** AltMedicine.com *** PeopleSuccess.com
*** HumorMatters.com *** SleepFoundation.org ***
BetterSleep.org *** Mind-Body.org *** Chopra.com (19)
TNP.com (Natural Pharmacist - 16) *** Abraham-Hicks.com (11)
*** HeartMath.com (10)

Special Events/Programs
AmericanHeart.org/HeartWalk/ ***
NIH.gov/nia/health/pubs/nasa-exercise (National Institute on
Aging's Exercise Guide) *** jiMotion.org (Joints in Motion
training team — arthritis) *** OneLife.AmericanHeart.org ***
WalkSport.com (mall walking program) *** Fitness.gov
(Presidential Sports Award for *all ages*) *** TheSparkPlan.com
(one of the Eight That Work) *** AgeMatters.com ***
CharitySports.org (for information on charity races across the
country to benefit a favorite cause) *** WeightWatchers.com
(33) *** AmericanHeart.org/HeartWalk/ (30) *** About.com
(click on fitness/wellness — 4) *** RunForLungs.com

Product & Sales
BreakAwayBooks.com *** chpOnLine.com (heart rate
monitors — plus) *** Homedics.com (wellness) *** Awards.com
(ribbons, trophies, ...) *** DougGrant.com (health) ***
Extique.com (Natural Hormonal Enhancement) ***
WheatGrass.com (nutrition) *** GreenFoods.com (Jerry Dunn
supplement) *** ClubCyrus.com/health/index.html (nutrition)
*** SwansonVitamins.com *** UltraFit-Endurance.com ***
Melissas.com (exotic produce plus) *** gaiam.com (Tai Chi) ***
SportsMusic.com *** DragonDoor.com (Tai Chi, Qigong, martial
arts) *** Chi-swingMachine.com *** Kashi.com (cereal plus) ***
SilkIsSoy.com (soymilk plus) *** Veat.com (Vegetarian "meat")
*** MedGraphics.com (MAXVO2)

Ed Mayhew with Mary Mayhew

References

Introduction
1. Gover J E. "The Fix Cannot Be Made In Small Doses." February, 2001. <www.todaysengineer.org>.
2. www.chopra.com
3. Nelson M E. "Vibrant Aging Overview - Your Virtual Trainer." <www.strongwomen.com/com/vibrant_aging>.
4. *The Wayne Dyer Info Page* - <http://grape.epix.net/~amigo000/dyer_home.html>.
5. Colarossi G. "American Fitness." *In the News - Age Fit.* 1/1/00 <www.ahealthyme.com>.
6. Stone K. "Mile Marker." 7/28/01 <www.uniontrib.com/sports/>.
7. Faigin R. *Natural Hormonal Enhancement.* Cedar Mountain: Extique Publisher, 2000.

Chapters 2 & 3 If They Can Do It ...
1. Benyo R, editor, McNelly D, Reese P, Ruettiger R, Wolff T L. *Marathon & Beyond.* Champaign: 42K(+) Press, Inc., Sept/Oct 2000 — Vol. 4, Issue 5.
2. Robinson R. "Masters of the Marathon." *Marathon & Beyond,* March/April 2000 — Vol 2, Issue 2.
3. Udesky L. "Seniors and Dance: Swinging After 60." 3/28/01 <www.ahealthyme.com>.
4. Kislevitz G W. *It's Never Too Late.* Halcottville: Breakaway Books, 2000.
5. Nelson M E. *Strong Women Stay Young.* New York: Bantam Books, 1997.
6. Benyo R. *Running Past 50.* Champaign: Human Kinetics, 1998.
7. Press clippings on Dick Collins courtesy of Ruth Anderson — 5/14/01.
8. Dyer W, Siegel B. Two articles. *World's Greatest Treasury of Health Secrets..* Bottom Line Books, 2000.
9. www.waynedyer.com
10. Chowka P B. Bernie Siegel March 1997 interview with Peter Barry Chowka (published in Nutrition Science News).

11. Arfaras F M. "Age Isn't Just A Candle On Your Birthday Cake." World Triathlon Corp., Inc., 2000 <www.ironmanlive.com>.
12. Arfaras F M, Autorino E, Brockenbrough R, Clark R. "A Lifestyle For A Champion."; "You Just Do It!"; "50's Family Man Now An Ironman, *Too.*"; "This Professed "Geezer" Athlete Is Having The Time Of His Life!". <www.ironmanlive.com>.
13. "At 50+ They (Still) Got Game." *USA Weekend* insert-magazine, March 16-18, 2000.
14. Carl Kristenson interview, winter 2000-2001 (E-mail, telephone and written letter correspondence).
15. Payton Jordan correspondence (personal letter, post card, and press clippings).
16. Janet Murray interview (E-mail correspondence and telephone - 2/5/01 & 12/01).
17. Sloan J. *Staying Fit Over Fifty.* Seattle: The Mountaineers Publication, 1999.
18. June Tatro telephone interview, 2/10/01.
19. "Australian Sets World 6 Day Record." <www.coolrunning.com.au/ultra/199804.shtml>.
20. Hawaiian Ironman Triathlon on ABC's Wide World of Sports, Spring, 1999.
21. Evelyn Tucci (82-year-old golfer's two holes-in-one) <cnnsi.com> — *Golf Plus.* 2/14/01; Jim Vance, News4 at 6 (Wash. D.C.), 2/15/01.
22. Portz-Shovlin E, ed. "Gene Gerow and Blanche McNutt, The Human Race." *Runner's World*, Emmaus: Rodale Press, April, 2000.
23. Biographies of master swimmers Sally Scott, Jean Durston, Anna Bauscher, Peter Jurczyk, Dave Malbrough, Walter Pfeiffer, Mildred Anderson, Aldo DaRosa, Lavelle Stoinoff, G. Harold "Gus" Langner, and Aileen Riggin Soule. <www.swimgold.org>.
24. Lucero A F. "Up, Up, And Away: 86 floors in 15 minutes." Sept/Oct 1999. <www.aarp.org>.
25. Scimone C. "Talk Test." *Runner's World* magazine. Emmaus: Rodale Press, May 2001.
26. "Speed Steps To Fitness - News For Healthy Living." *Health magazine*, September 1998.

27. Warren Utes telephone interview, 1/15/01 (Norm Green E-mail, 11/18/00).
28. Norm Green E-mail interviews starting 11/18/01.
29. Robinson R. "Masters of the Marathon." *Marathon & Beyond.* Champaign: 42K(+) Press, Inc., March/April 1998, Vol. 2, Issue 2.
30. James Hill interviews (E-mail & telephone starting 11/00).
31. "Wear-Tester Profile: James Hill." *Runner's World magazine.* Emmaus: Rodale Press.
32. Helen Klein interviews (Phone and mail starting 11/27/00).
33. Anderson S L. *Helen Klein: No Limits Living,* Folsom: SLA Associates.
34. Kislevitz G W. *It's Never Too Late.* Halcottsville: Breakaway Books, 2000.
35. Benyo R. *Running Past 50.* Champaign: Human Kinetics, 1998.
36. Denver Fox interviews (E-mail 10/28/00 & 10/29/00).
37. Ruth Anderson interviews (E-mails beginning 12/6/00).
38. Jerry Dunn interviews (E-mail correspondence beginning 12/22/00).
39. Ruibal S. Jerry Dunn articles: *USA Today*, Fall, 2000 and some at <www.marathonman.org>.
40. Kahn R L, Rowe J W. *Successful Aging.* and Dell Trade Paperback, 1998.
41. Dreyfuss I. "Studies: Older Exercisers Are Able To Gain Strength." *The Winchester Star*, 10/21/00.
42. "Tough Enough." *Modern Maturity magazine.* AARP publication, Sept/Oct 2000.
43. www.strongwomen.com
44. Life J. "Ask Dr. Life." *MuscleMedia magazine.* Golden: Muscle Media Publications, Jan/Feb 2001.
45. Wibecan K. "Body By Jim." *Modern Maturity magazine*, July/August 1998.
46. Noland D. "Life's A Beach." *Modern Maturity*, Mar/Apr 2001.
47. www.surfingforlife.com
48. Jean Sterling E-mail interview — 10/29/00.

49. King J. "Sailor beats the sea and gets a hero's welcome." *South Florida Sun-Sentinel,* 12/8/01 <SunSentinel.com>.
50. "John Keston: Master Blaster." *Runner's World.* Emmaus: Rodale Press, February 2002.

Chapter 4 Minding Your Own Business
1. "The Mind Trick That Replaces Exercise." staff. *Woman's World magazine,* Spring 2001.
2. Hicks J, Hicks E. *A New Beginning I.* San Antonio: Abraham-Hicks Publications, 1988.
3. www.Abraham-Hicks.com
4. "Overcoming Fear of Failure." Editors. *World's Greatest Treasury ofHealth Secrets.* Bottom Line Books, 2000.
5. *Modern Maturity magazine.* Jan/Feb 2001.
6. *Journal of the American Geriatrics Society.* Vol. 47, No. 11.
7. "The Power of Laughter." <www.thriveonline.oxygen.com>.
8. "Humor Therapy." <www.ahealthyme.com/topic/humor>.
9. Wooten P. "Jest For the Health of It! — 'Humor Skills ....'" <www.jesthealth.com>.
10. Medinger J. "Dick Collins 1933 - 1997. *Ultra Running,* April 1997.

Chapter 5 Researchers Stumble Upon the Fountain of Youth
1. Kislevitz G W. *It's Never Too Late.* Halscottville: Breakaway Books, 2000.
2. Nelson M E. "Vibrant Aging Overview." 3/25/01 <www.strongwomen.com>.
3. Lindeman B. "In Your Prime," *Winchester Star,* 2/3/01.
4. "Finding the Fountain of Youth." Editors. *The World's Treasury of Health Secrets.* Bottom Line Books, 2000.
5. Nelson M E. *Strong Women Stay Young.* New York: Bantam Trade Paperback, 1997.
6. Ibid. Your Virtual Trainer with Miriam E. Nelson, Ph.D. <www.strongwomen.com>.

7. National Library of Medicine, Jan./Feb. 1999. (*New England Journal of Medicine* 338:94, 1998) <www.drmcdougall.com>.

8. "Longevity News." *Medicine and Science in Sports and Exercise.* 2000; 32:2005 - 2011. <www.worldhealth.net>.

9. Dougherty K, Gaesser G A.. *The Spark.* New York: Simon and Schuster, 2001.

10. Miller K E. "Is Aerobic Training In COPD Patients Safe And Effective?" *American Family Physician* (6/15/00) - *Arch. Phys. Med. Rehabilitation,* Jan. 2000; 81: 102 - 9. <www.healthyme.com>.

11. Woolston C. "Seniors and Weightlifting." <www.healthyme.com>.

12. "Ten Exercise Myths." *Nutrition Action Healthletter.* 1/1/00 <www.ahealthyme.com>.

13. Billingsley J. "Living Longer and Loving It." 3/28/01 <www.ahealthyme.com>.

14. Conway C. "You Won't Believe What's In Your Sweat." <http://member.compuserve.com/new/html/fte/2k/3.html>.

15. Haas F. "Exercise Is Good For Asthmatics." *The World's Treasury ofHealth Secrets.* Bottom Line Books, 2000.

16. Minor M. "Anti-Arthritis Exercise." *The World's Treasury of Health Secrets.* Bottom Line Books, 2000.

17. "Longevity News — World Health Network." 5/31/00 <www.onhealth.com>. (The official site of the American Academy of Anti-Aging).

18. Foreyt J. "Exercise Beats Dieting." *The World's Treasury of Health Secrets.* Bottom Line Books, 2000.

19. Lee K. "Working Up A Good Appetite." *Health magazine,* Oct. 1998.

20. *Prevention magazine,* March, 2001.

21. "Save Up To $1,053 A Year!" *Prevention,* March, 2001.

22. "Lower Direct Medical Costs Associated With Physical Activity." 12/14/00 <www.cdc.gov>.

23. Vann K. "Mature Years." *Winchester Star,* 5/19/01.

Chapter 6 Sustenance Abuse

1. Yeager S. *The Doctors' Book of Food Remedies.* Emmaus: Rodale, Inc., 1998.

2. Payton Jordan — personal correspondence, Fall, 2000.
3. Ruth Anderson — E-mail correspondence, 12/6/00.
4. Warren Utes — Telephone interviews, 1/15/01 & 12/01.
5. Carl Kristenson — personal correspondence (letter), 12/7/00.
6. June Tatro — telephone interview, 2/10/01.
7. James Hill — E-mail correspondence, 11/21/00.
8. Jerry Dunn — E-mail correspondence, 1/9/01 & 1/11/01.
9. Helen Klein — Telephone interviews, 11/27/00 & 12/19/01.
10. Mayhew E. *Winchester Wellness Tip*, 7/97.
11. Editors. *Eat and Heal.* Peachtree City: F C & A Publishing, 2001.
12. "Lower Cancer Risk: Eat What?" *What's New On Compuserve.* <www.member.compuserve.com, 5/13/01>.
13. *American Institute for Cancer Research Newsletter.* Issue 71, Spring 2001.
14. Cooper B. "Master Blaster." *Runner's World.* Emmaus: Rodale, Inc., August 2001.
15. "USDA Food Guide Pyramid." <www.idd-inc.com/pyramidtracker/>.
16. *Men's Fitness magazine*, May 2001.
17. "The Proven Way To Lose Weight. *Health magazine*, October, 1998.
18. Life J. "Performance Nutrition." *Muscle Media*, July/August 2001.
19. Faigin R. *Natural Hormonal Enhancement.* Cedar Mountain: Extique Publishing, 2000.
20. Mayhew E. *The Skinny Book of Fat.* Winchester: Just Ducky Books (self published), 1997.
21. Wibecan K. "Body By Jim." *Modern Maturity,* July/August, 1998.
22. "The Amazing Peanut Butter Diet." *Prevention magazine*, March 2001.
23. Editors. *Eat and Heal.* Peachtree City: FC&A Medical Publishers, 2001.
24. Smith C M. "Don't Forget About Nutrition." *On Site Fitness*, Jan./Feb., 2000.

25. "Smoking Accelerates the Aging Process." *Health Scout*, 9/6/00.
26. Lee K. "Peanut Power." *Health*, Sept. 1998.
27. "High Fiber Diet." *New England Journal Of Medicine*, Vol. 342, No. 19.
28. Ross E. "Study Says Daily Soda Can Make Kids Fat." 2/16/01 <www.tcpalm.com>.
29. *Water for Life Newsletter,* Viva Healing Arts Center. <www.vivahealingarts.com>.
30. Vann K. "Drinking Plenty of Water Important In Winter." *The Hartford Courant*, May 2001.

Chapter 7 The 60-Second Solution
1. www.freeze-framer.com
2. Childre D L. *Cut Thru.* Boulder Creek: Planetary Publications, 1996.
3. "How To Use Guided Imagery for Wellness."*World's Greatest Treasury of Health Secrets.* Bottom Line Books, 2000.
4. Editors. "The Mind Trick That Replaces Exercise." *Woman's World*, 4/1/01.
5. Benson H. "20 Minutes A Day To A Much Happier, Much Healthier You." *World's Greatest Treasury of Health Secrets.* Bottom Line Books, 2000.
6. Conroy C. "Scientific PROOF That Prayer Works!?" 12/26/01. <http://member.compuserve.com/new/html/fte/2k/7.html>.
7. McCraty R. "Music And the Immune System." 1999 <www.heartmath.org/researchpapers>.
8. Chopra D. *Perfect Health.* New York: Harmony Books, 1991.
9. Conroy C. "Ha! Ha! Ha! Laughing Does What?" 5/30/01 <www.member.compuserve.com>.
10. Fryon W. "The Healing Effects of Humor." <www.thriveonline.oxygen.com>.
11. "Humor Therapy." 5/13/01 <www.ahealthyme.com>.
12. "Study Says 25 Died From Long Flights." Reuters. 12/28/00 <www.dailynews.yahoo.com>.
13. Editors. "Cadio Training For Fat Burning." *Total Training Guide 2000.* Muscle Media, 2/1/01.

14. Maffetone P. *The Maffetone Method.* Camden: McGraw Hill, 2000.

Chapter 8 Eight That Work
1. Nelson M E. *Strong Women Stay Young.* New York: Bantam Books, 1997.
2. www.strongwomen.com (success stories).
3. Phillips B. *Body For Life.* New York: Harper Collins Publisher, 1999.
4. *Body For Life Challenge 2001* (instructional booklet).
5. Cole A. "Before and After." *Modern Maturity,* Sept./Oct. 2000.
6. Editors. *Total Training Guide.* Muscle Media, January 2001.
7. McDougall J A.. *The McDougall Program.* New York: A Plume Book, 1991.
8. www.drmcdougall.com
9. www.cooperaerobics.com/tip_walkforlife.htm
10. www.cooperaerobics.com
11. Maffetone P. *The Maffetone Method.* Camden: Ragged Mountain Press/McGraw Hill, 2000.
12. Mittleman S. *Slow Burn.* New York: Harper Collins, 2000.
13. Childre D L. *Cut Thru.* Boulder Creek: Planetary Publications, 1996.
14. Beech D, Childre D, Martin H. *The HeartMath Solution.* New York: HarperSanFrancisco, 1999.
15. www.heartmath.org/researchpapers/abstracts/ab2.html
16. www.thesparkplan.com
17. Dougherty K, Gaessar G A.. *The Spark.* New York: Simon & Schuster, 2001.
18. www.diabetes.org/teamdiabetes/team3/
19. Team Diabetes literature kit.

Chapter 9 Fitter After 50 Hits Home
1. "Protein Supplements." 3/31/01 <www.ahealthyme.com>.
2. Editors. *ProSource Buyer's Guide 2001.* 1-800-310-1555.
3. *Sports Supplement Review, 3rd edition.* Bill Phillips. Golden: Mile High Publishing.
4. Cooper K. Notes from Dr. Kenneh Cooper's interview on the G. Gordon Liddy radio show, 4/12/01.

5. Cooper K. "Anti-Aging Supplements." *World's Greatest Treasury of Health Secrets.* Bottom Line Books, 2000.
6. *VitaMix* brochure, 2000. 1-800-848-2649.
7. www.freeze-framer.com
8. "Sports Breather." <www.j-f-financial.com/sportsbreather>.
9. *Total Gym exercise system Owner's Manual.* Fitness Quest, Inc., 1999.
10. www.totalgym.com
11. Randy Wingfield interview — 11/017/01
12. Ray Kitchen telephone interview — 11/22/01
13. Burr Grim interview — 11/17/01
14. Jason Paige interview — 11/17/01
15. Chuck Raper interview — 11/17/01
16. Kathy Smart telephone interview — 11/22/01
17. Sandy Adams telephone interview — 11/23/01
18. Pat Rice interview — 11/28/01

Ed Mayhew with Mary Mayhew

Index

Due to frequent first-name reference to featured Masters of Fitness, individual are alphabetically indexed by first name

ABOUT THE AUTHOR

Ed Mayhew is the author of *Educating Your Star Child, The Skinny Book of Fat,* and *The Important Journey* (audiocassette). A professional educator for thirty-five years, he has specialized in physical fitness for children. As he crossed the half-century mark, he turned his attention to adult fitness issues. Ed is an avid runner, a cyclist, sports enthusiast, and definitely fitter after 50. He is married to his co-author, Mary.

Note: For *Fitter After 50*, Mayhew conducted dozens of interviews with the Masters of Fitness – the real authors of much of *FA50*'s insights and inspiration – and researched dozens more to glean their secrets and share them with you.

Mary Mayhew has authored two other books: *Your Star Child* (nonfiction) and *Great Adventure: A Coming of Age at Going on Fifty* (a novel). She is also the co-author of *Educating Your Star Child.* Besides writing, Mary is an artist, musician, and mother of the Mayhews' two daughters, Catherine and Joanna. She illustrated the covers and/or "innards" of most of the above-mentioned books, including *FA50*.

www.FitterAfter50.com

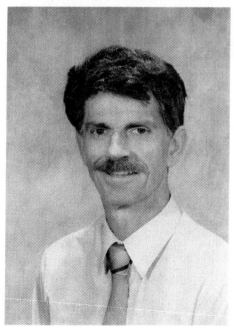

Printed in the United States
146465LV00002B/22/A

9 781403 302571